# The Vibrant Keto Air Fryer Recipe Book

Super Fast  and Delicious   Seafood Recipes to boost your health

River Hunt

# Introduction

What's the difference between an air fryer and deep fryer? Air fryers bake food at a high temperature with a high-powered fan, while deep fryers cook food in a vat of oil that has been heated up to a specific temperature. Both cook food quickly, but an air fryer requires practically zero preheat time while a deep fryer can take upwards of 10 minutes. Air fryers also require little to no oil and deep fryers require a lot that absorb into the food. Food comes out crispy and juicy in both appliances, but don't taste the same, usually because deep fried foods are coated in batter that cook differently in an air fryer vs a deep fryer. Battered foods needs to be sprayed with oil before cooking in an air fryer to help them color and get crispy, while the hot oil soaks into the batter in a deep fryer. Flour-based batters and wet batters don't cook well in an air fryer, but they come out very well in a deep fryer.

The ketogenic diet is one such example. The diet calls for a very small number of carbs to be eaten. This means food such as rice, pasta, and other starchy vegetables like potatoes are off the menu. Even relaxed versions of the keto diet minimize carbs to a large extent and this compromises the goals of many dieters. They end up having to exert large amounts of willpower to follow the diet. This doesn't do them any favors since willpower is like a muscle. At some point, it tires and this is when the dieter goes right back to their old pattern of eating. I have personal experience with this. In terms of health benefits, the keto diet offers the most. The reduction of carbs forces your body to mobilize fat and this results in automatic fat loss and better health.

Feel free to mix and match the recipes you see in here and play around with them. Eating is supposed to be fun! Unfortunately, we've associated fun eating with unhealthy food. This doesn't have to be the case. The air fryer, combined with the Mediterranean diet, will make your mealtimes fun-filled again and full of taste. There's no grease and messy cleanups to deal with anymore. Are you excited yet?

You should be! You're about to embark on a journey full of air fried goodness!

# Table of Contents

# Sesame Prawns with Firecracker Sauce

**Cooking Time:**

20 minutes

**Servings:**4

**Ingredients:**

1 lb tiger prawns, peeled

Salt and black pepper to taste

2 eggs

½ cup flour

¼ cup sesame seeds

¾ cup seasoned breadcrumbs

**Firecracker sauce:**

⅓ cup sour cream

2 tbsp buffalo sauce

¼ cup spicy ketchup

1 green onion, chopped

**Directions:**

1.Preheat air fryer to 390 F. Beat the eggs in a bowl with salt. In another bowl, mix breadcrumbs with sesame seeds.

2.In a third bowl, mix flour with salt and pepper. Dip prawns in the flour and then in the eggs, and finally in the crumbs.

3.Spray with cooking spray and Air Fryer for 10 minutes, flipping once. Meanwhile, mix well all thee sauce ingredients, except for green onion in a bowl.

4.Serve the prawns with firecracker sauce and scatter with freshly chopped green onions.

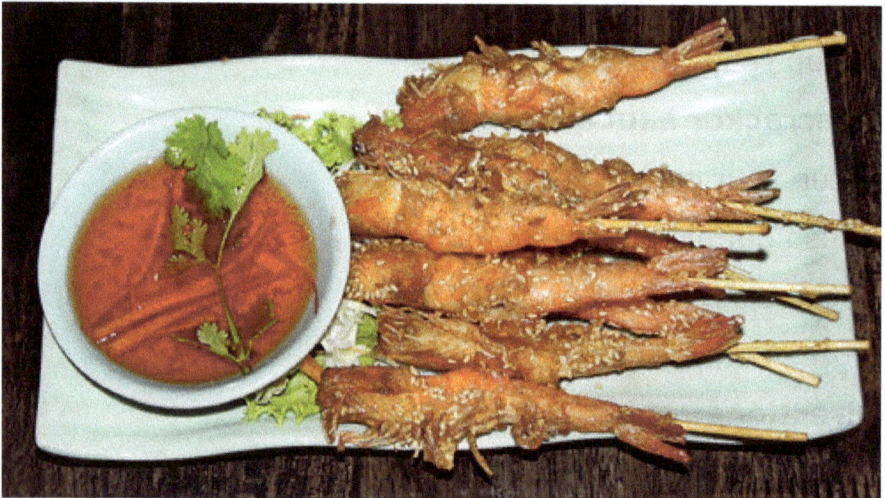

# Wild Salmon with Creamy Parsley Sauce

**Cooking Time:**

20 minutes

**Servings:**4

**Ingredients:**

4 Alaskan wild salmon fillets
2 tsp olive oil
Salt to taste
½ cup heavy cream
½ cup milk
2 tbsp fresh parsley, chopped

**Directions:**

1.Preheat air fryer to 380 F. Drizzle the fillets with olive oil, and season with salt and black pepper. Place salmon in the frying basket and Bake for 15 minutes, turning once until tender and crispy.

2.In a bowl, mix milk, parsley, salt, and whipped cream. Serve the salmon with the sauce.

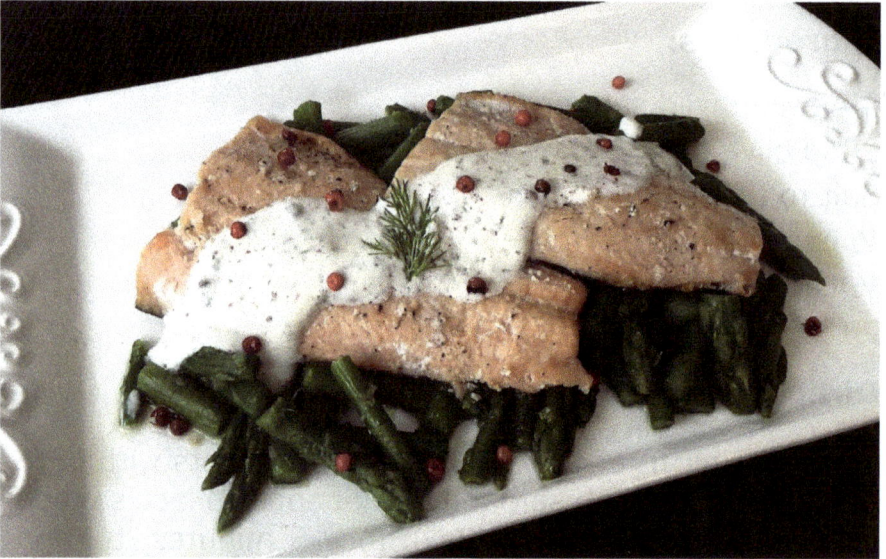

# Fried Catfish Fillets

**Cooking Time:**

20 minutes

**Servings:**4

**Ingredients:**

2 catfish fillets

½ cup breadcrumbs

¼ tsp cayenne pepper

¼ tsp fish seasoning

1 tbsp fresh parsley, chopped

Salt to taste

**Directions:**

1.Preheat air fryer to 400 F. Pour all the dry ingredients, except for the parsley, in a bowl. Add in the fish pieces and toss to coat.


2.Lightly spray the fish with olive oil. Put the fillets in the fryer basket and Air Fryer for 6-7 minutes. Flip and cook further for 5 minutes. Garnish with freshly chopped parsley and serve.

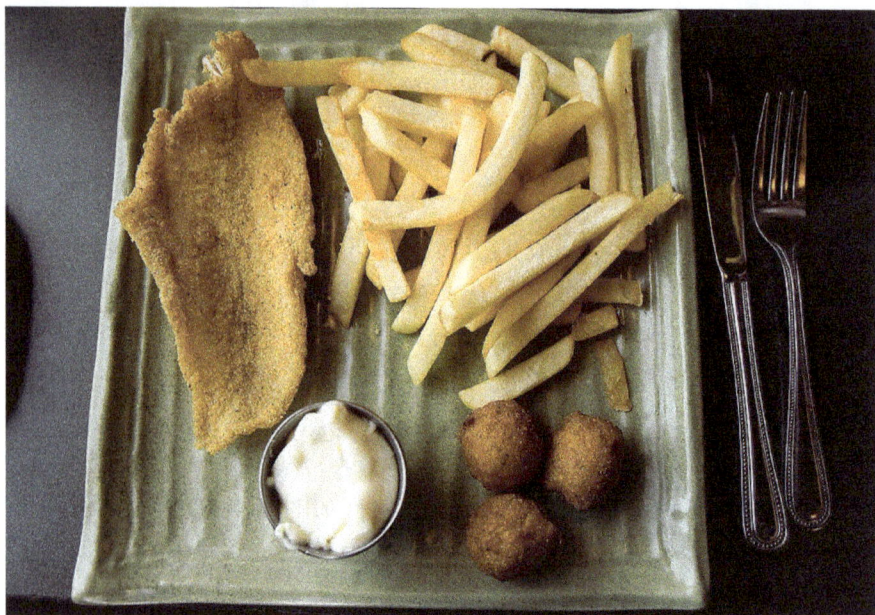

# Barramundi Fillets in Lemon Sauce

**Cooking Time:**

30 minutes

**Servings:**4

**Ingredients:**

4 barramundi fillets

1 lemon, juiced

Salt and black pepper to taste

2 tbsp butter

½ cup white wine

8 black peppercorns

2 cloves garlic, minced

2 shallots, chopped

**Directions:**

1.Preheat air fryer to 390 F. Season the fillets with salt and pepper. Place in the greased air fryer basket.

2.AirFryer for 15 minutes, flipping once halfway through until the edges are golden brown. Remove to a plate. Melt the butter in a pan over low heat. Add in garlic and shallots and stir-fry for 3 minutes.

4.Pour in white wine, lemon juice, and peppercorns. Cook until the liquid is reduced by three quarters, about 3-5 minutes. Adjust the seasoning and strain the sauce. Drizzle the sauce over the fish and serve.

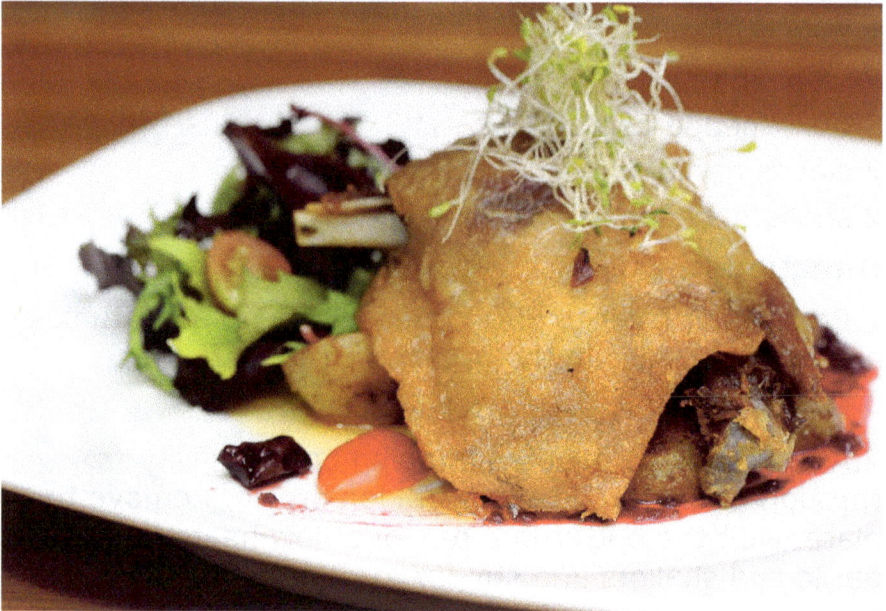

# Peach Salsa & Beer Halibut Tacos

**Cooking Time:**

15 minutes

**Servings:**4

**Ingredients:**

4 corn tortillas

1 halibut fillet

2 tbsp olive oil

1 ½ cups flour

1 can beer

A pinch of salt

4 tbsp peach salsa

4 tsp fresh cilantro, chopped

1 tsp baking powder

**Directions:**

1.Preheat air fryer to 390 F. In a bowl, combine flour, baking powder, and salt.

2.Pour in some of the beer, enough to form a batter-like consistency. Save the rest of the beer to gulp with the tacos. Slice the fillet into 4 strips.

3.Dip them into the beer batter and arrange on a lined baking dish. Place in the fryer and Air Fryer for 8 minutes. Spread the peach salsa on the tortillas. Top with fish strips and cilantro to serve.

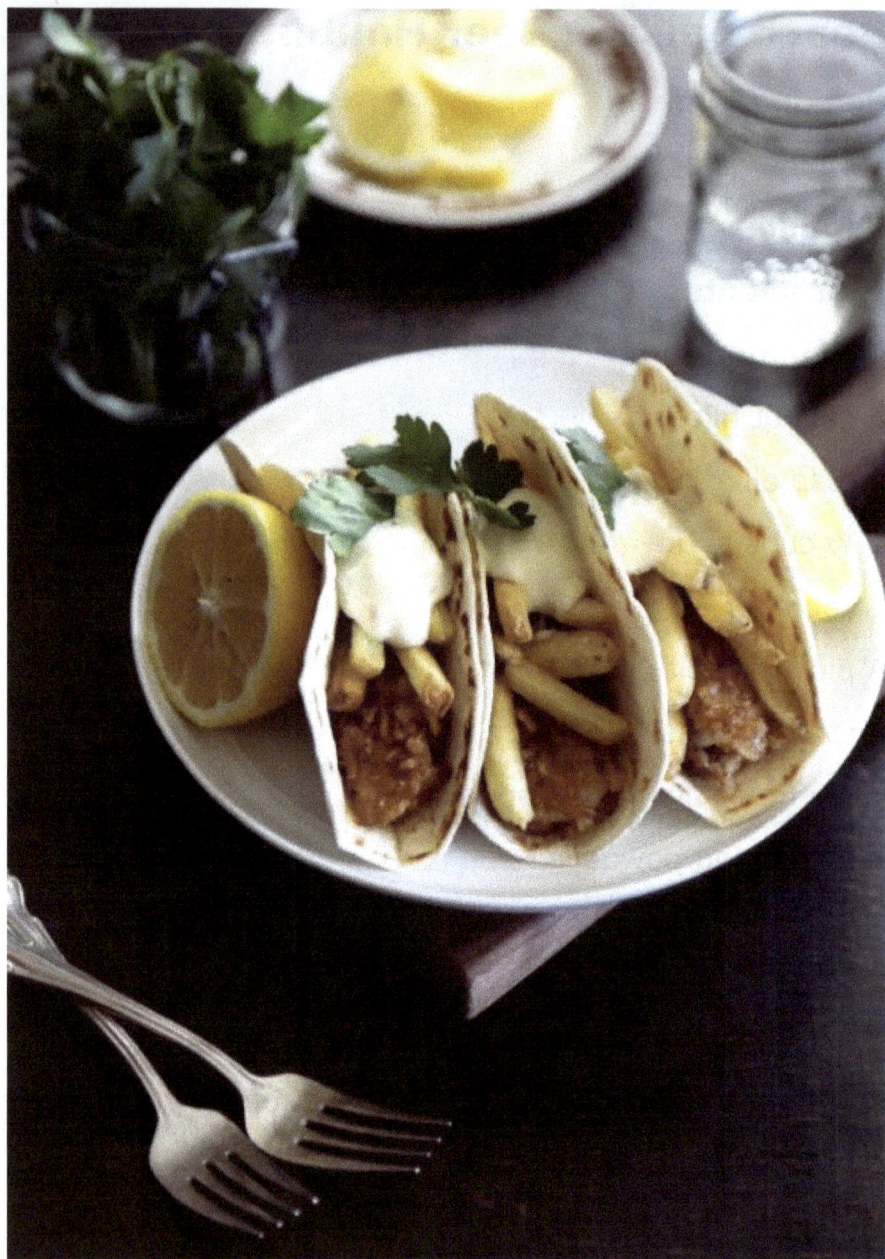

# Crab Fritters with Sweet Chili Sauce

**Cooking Time:**

20 minutes

**Servings:**4

**Ingredients:**

1 lb jumbo crabmeat

1 lime, zested and juiced

1 tsp ginger paste

1 tsp garlic puree

1 tbsp fresh cilantro, chopped

1 red chili, roughly chopped

1 egg

¼ cup panko breadcrumbs

1 tsp soy sauce sauce

3 tbsp sweet chili sauce

**Directions:**

1.Preheat air fryer to 400 F. In a bowl, mix crabmeat, lime zest, egg, ginger paste, and garlic puree. Form small cakes out of the mixture and dredge them into breadcrumbs.

2.Place in the greased frying basket and Air Fryer for 15 minutes, shaking once until golden. In a small bowl, mix the sweet chili sauce with lime juice and soy sauce.

3.Serve the fritters topped with cilantro and sweet chili sauce

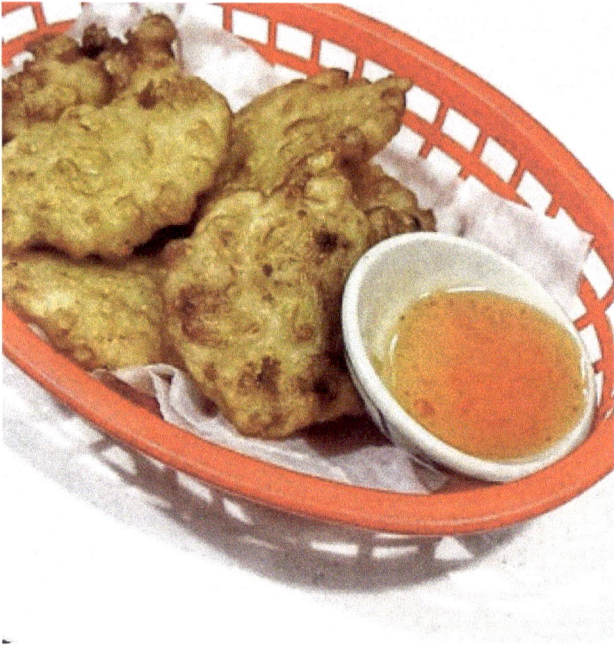

# Ale-Battered Scampi with Tartare Sauce

**Cooking Time:**

15 minutes

**Servings:** 4

**Ingredients:**

1 lb prawns, peeled and deveined

1 cup plain flour

1 cup ale beer

Salt and black pepper to taste

Tartare sauce:

½ cup mayonnaise

2 tbsp capers, roughly chopped

2 tbsp fresh dill, chopped

1 pickled cucumber, finely chopped

2 tsp lemon juice

½ tsp Worcestershire sauce

**Directions:**

1.Preheat air fryer to 380 F. In a bowl, mix all the sauce ingredients and keep in the fridge. Mix flour, ale beer, salt, and pepper in a large bowl.

2.Dip in the prawns and place them in the frying basket. Air Fryer for 10 minutes, shaking halfway through the cooking time. Serve with the tartare sauce.

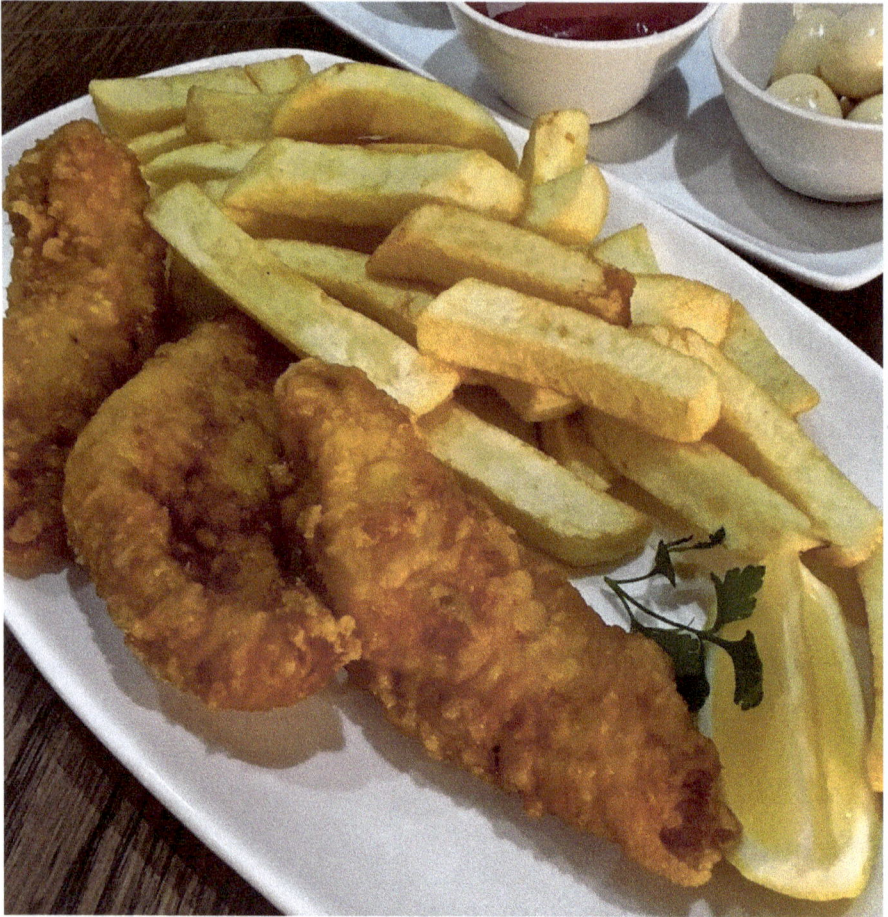

# Herbed Garlic Lobster

**Cooking Time:**

30 minutes

**Servings:**4

**Ingredients:**

4 oz lobster tails, halved

1 garlic clove, minced

1 tbsp butter

Salt and black pepper to taste

½ tbsp lemon Juice

## Directions:

1.Blend all ingredients, except for lobster, in a food processor.

2.Clean the skin of the lobster and cover it with the mixture.

3.Preheat air fryer to 380 F. Place the lobster in the frying basket and Air Fry for 10 minutes, turning once halfway through. Serve with fresh herbs.

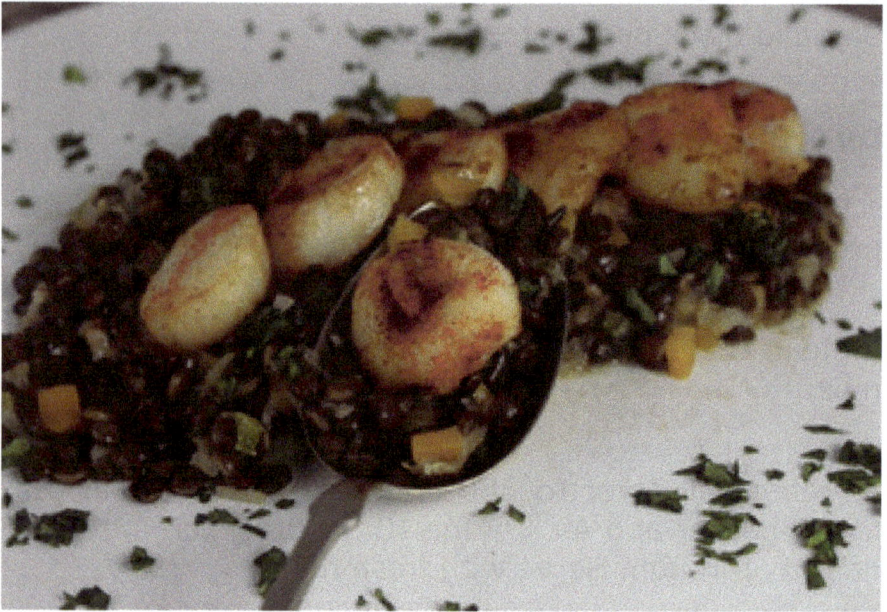

# Soy sauce glazed

**Cook Time:**

15 minutes
**Servings:**4
**Ingredients:**

2 cod fillets

1 tbsp olive oil Salt and black pepper to taste

1 tbsp soy sauce

1 tbsp sesame oil

¼ tsp ginger powder

¼ tsp honey

**Directions:**

1.Preheat air fryer to 370 F. In a bowl, combine olive oil, salt, and pepper. Rub the mixture onto the fillets. Place them on a piece of aluminum sheet and then in the greased frying basket.

2.Bake for 6 minutes. Meanwhile, combine the soy sauce, ginger powder, honey, and sesame oil in a small bowl.

3.Flip the fillets and brush them with the glaze. Cook for 3 more minutes. Serve warm.

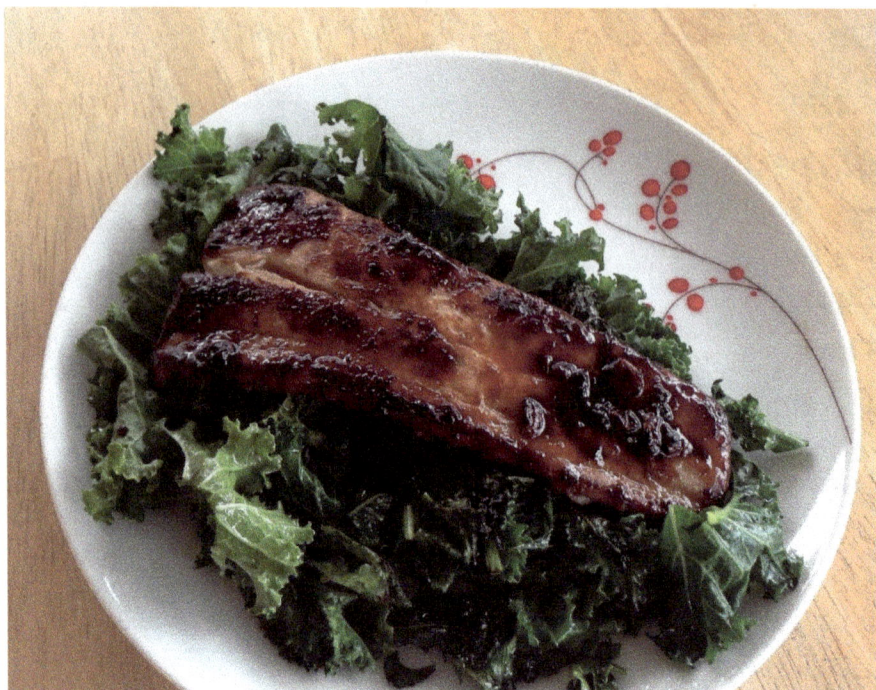

# Pistachio-Crusted Salmon Fillets

**Cooking Time:**

20 minutes

**Servings:**2

**Ingredients:**

2 salmon fillets

1 tsp mustard

4 tbsp pistachios, chopped

Salt and black pepper to taste

1 tsp garlic powder

2 tsp lemon juice

2 tbsp Parmesan cheese, grated

1 tsp olive oil

**Directions:**

1.Preheat air fryer to 350 F. Whisk together mustard, olive oil, lemon juice, salt, black pepper, and garlic powder in a bowl. Rub the mustard mixture onto salmon fillets.

2.Combine the pistachios with Parmesan cheese; sprinkle on top of the salmon.

3.Place the salmon in the greased frying basket, skin side down, and Bake for 12-13 minutes. Flip at the 7-minute mark. Serve.

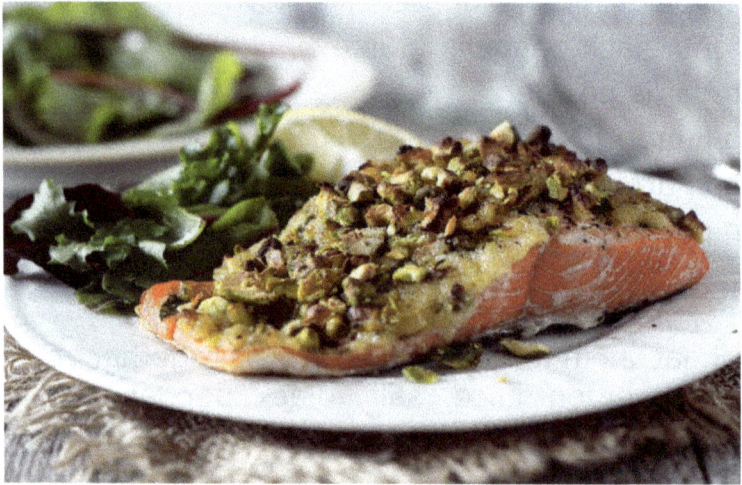

# Smoked Trout Frittata

**Cooking Time:**

20 minutes

**Servings:**2

**Ingredients:**

2 tbsp olive oil

1 onion, sliced

1 egg, beaten

6 tbsp crème fraiche

½ tbsp horseradish sauce

1 cup smoked trout, diced

2 tbsp fresh dill, chopped

**Directions:**

1.Preheat air fryer to 350 F. Heat olive oil in a pan over medium heat. Stir-fry onion for 3 minutes.

2.In a bowl, mix the egg with crème fraiche and horseradish sauce.

3.Add the onion, dill, and trout and mix well. Pour the mixture into a greased baking dish and Bake in the fryer for 14 minutes until golden

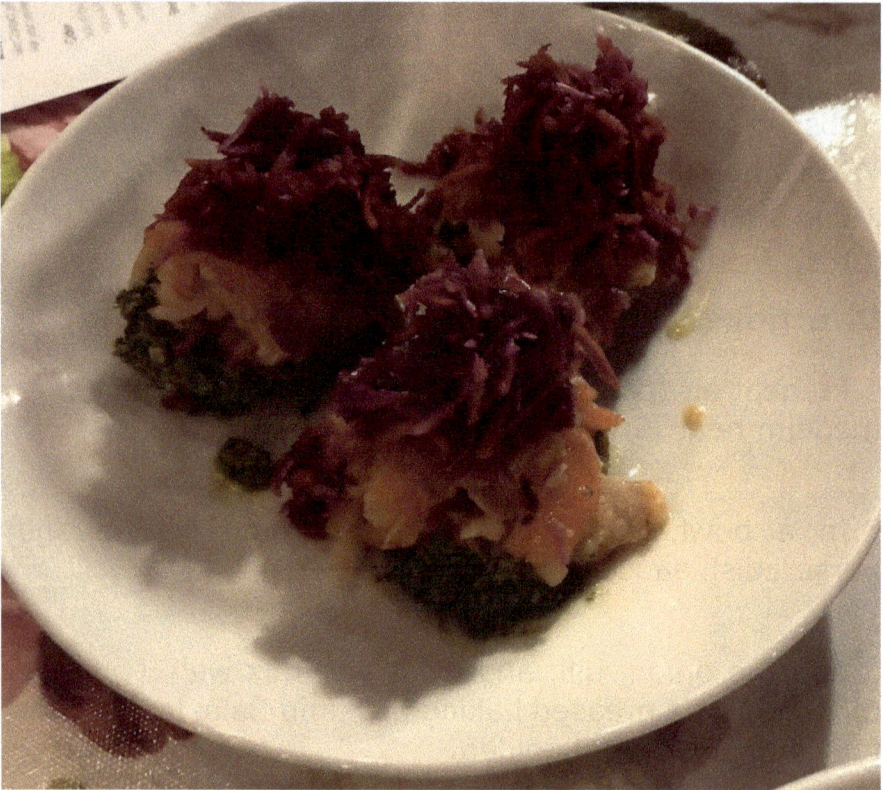

# Effortless Tuna Fritters

**Cook Time:**

20minutes

**Servings:**2

**Ingredients:**

5 oz canned tuna

1 tsp lime juice

½ tsp paprika

¼ cup flour

½ cup milk

1 small onion, diced

2 eggs

1 tsp chili powder, optional

½ tsp salt

**Directions:**

1.Place all ingredients in a bowl and mix well. Make two large patties out of the mixture. Refrigerate them for 30 minutes.

2.Then, remove and Air Fryer the patties for 13-15 minutes at 350 F in the greased frying basket, flipping once halfway through cooking. Serve warm

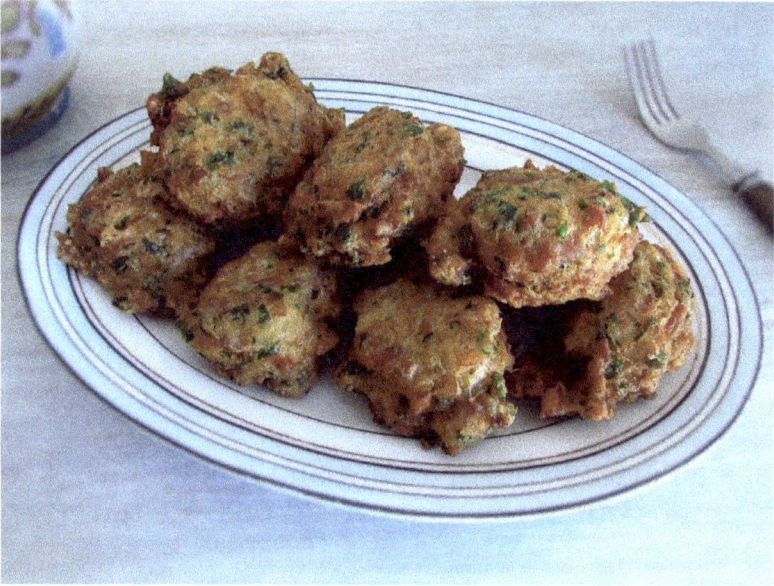

# Smoked Fish Quiche

**Cooking Time:**

15 minutes

**Servings:**3

**Ingredients:**

1 pie crust

5 eggs, lightly beaten

4 tbsp heavy cream

¼ cup green onions, finely chopped

2 tbsp fresh parsley, chopped

1 tsp baking powder

Salt and black pepper to taste

1 lb smoked salmon, chopped

1 cup mozzarella cheese,

shredded

**Directions:**

1.In a bowl, whisk eggs, heavy cream, green onions, parsley, baking powder, salt, and pepper. Stir in salmon and mozzarella cheese.

2.Roll out the pie crust and press it gently into a greased quiche pan that fits in your air fryer. Prick the pie all over with a fork.

3.Pour in the salmon mixture and place the pan inside the fryer. Bake for 25 minutes at 360 F. Let cool slightly before slicing.

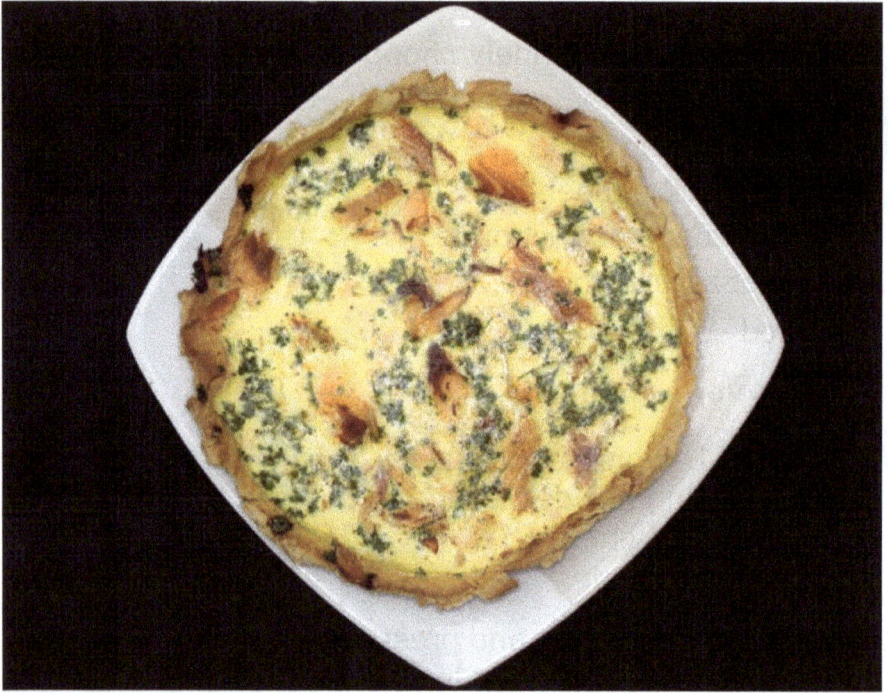

# Louisiana-Style Shrimp

## Cooking time:

15 minutes
**Servings:**4

## Ingredients:

1 lb shrimp, peeled and deveined

1 egg, beaten

1 cup flour

1 cup breadcrumbs

2 tbsp Cajun seasoning

Salt and black pepper to taste

1 lemon, cut into wedges

## Directions:

1.Preheat air fryer to 390 F. Spray the air fryer basket with cooking spray. Beat the eggs in a bowl and season with salt and black pepper.

2.In a separate bowl, mix breadcrumbs with Cajun seasoning. In a third bowl, pour the flour. Dip shrimp in flour, then in the eggs, and finally in the crumbs mixture.

3.Spray with cooking spray and Air Fryer in the frying basket for 5 minutes. Flip and cook for 4 more minutes. Serve with lemon wedges.

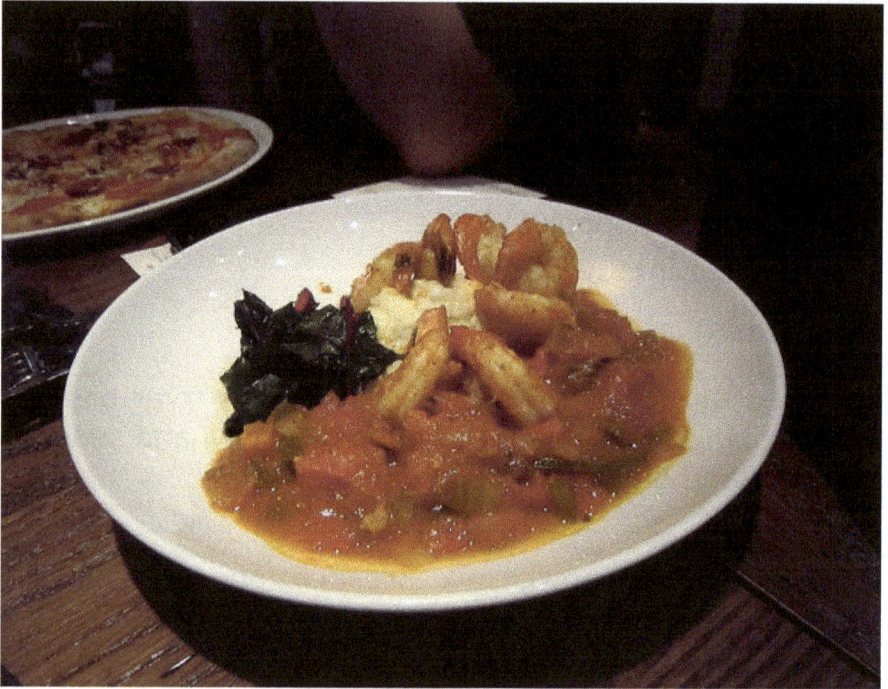

# Cajun-Rubbed Jumbo Shrimp

**Cooking Time:**

15 minutes

**Servings:**4

**Ingredients:**

1 lb jumbo shrimp, deveined

Salt to taste

¼ tsp old bay seasoning

⅓ tsp smoked paprika

¼ tsp cayenne pepper

1 tbsp olive oil

**Directions:**

1.Preheat air fryer to 390 degrees. In a bowl, add shrimp, paprika, olive oil, salt, old bay seasoning, and cayenne pepper; mix well.

2.Place the shrimp in the fryer and Air Fryer for 8-10 minutes, shaking once.

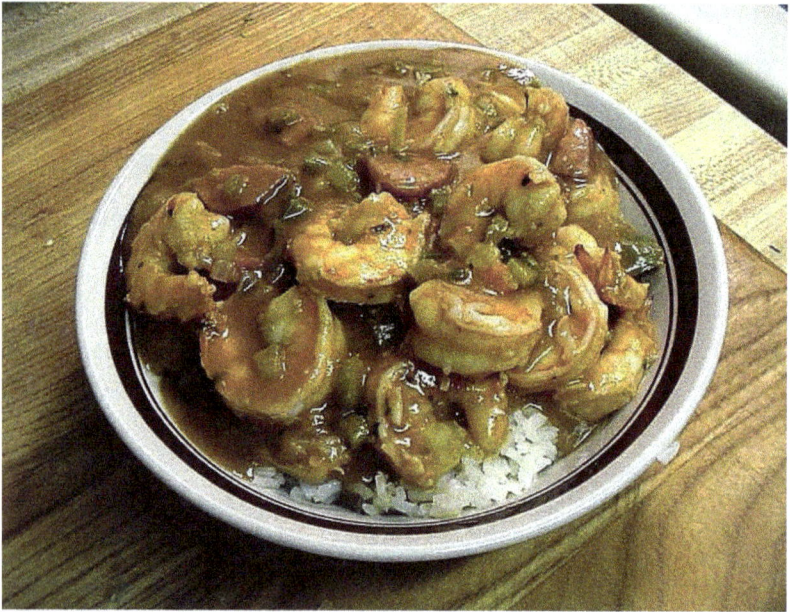

# Herbed Garlic Lobster

**Cooking Time:**

15 minutes

**Servings:**4

**Ingredients:**

4 oz lobster tails, halved

1 garlic clove, minced

1 tbsp butter

Salt and black pepper to taste

½ tbsp lemon Juice

**Directions:**

1.Blend all ingredients, except for lobster, in a food processor.


2.Clean the skin of the lobster and cover it with the mixture.


3.Preheat air fryer to 380 F. Place the lobster in the frying basket and Air Fryer for 10 minutes, turning once halfway through. Serve with fresh herbs. Enjoy!

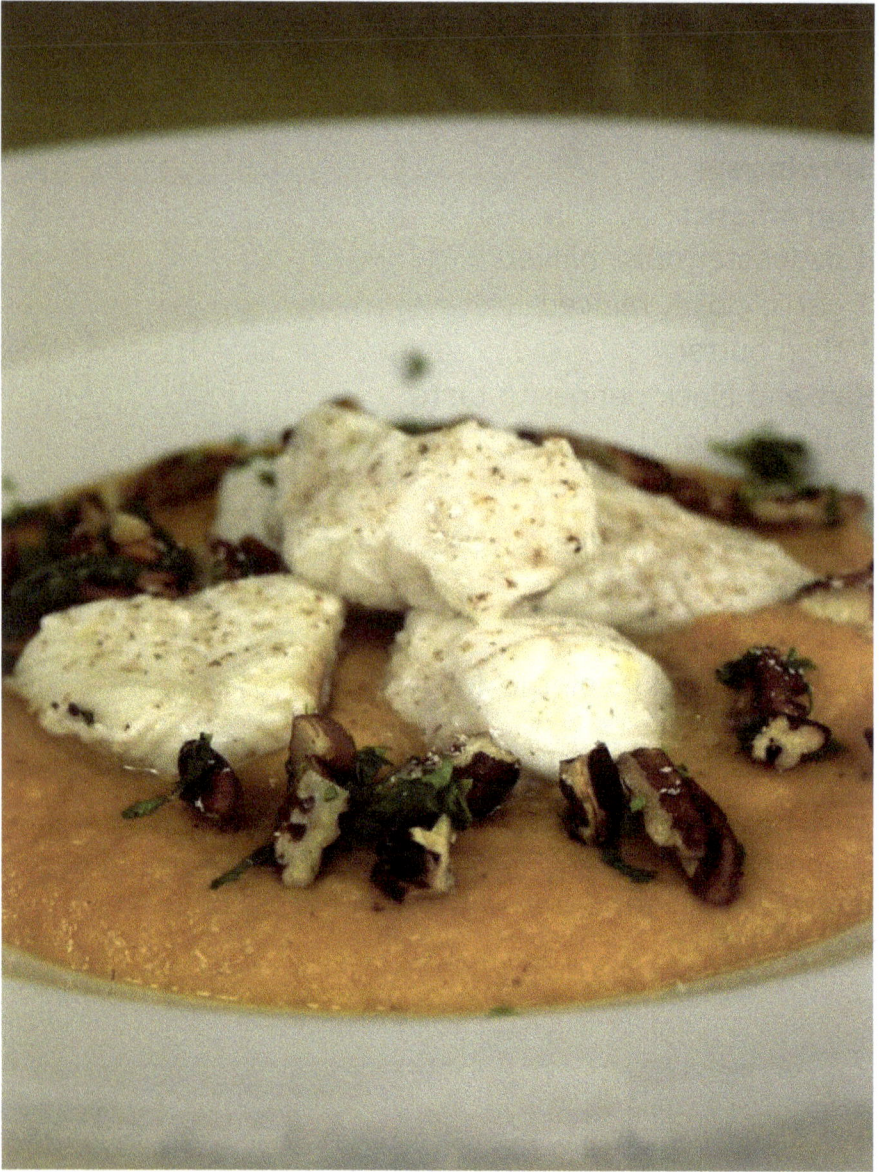

# Salmon Cakes

## Cooking Time:

15 minutes

## Servings:4

## Ingredients:

1 lb cooked salmon

4 potatoes, boiled and mashed

½ cup flour

2 tbsp capers, chopped

2 tbsp fresh parsley, chopped

1 tbsp olive oil Zest of

1 lemon

## Directions:

1.Place mashed potatoes in a bowl and flake the salmon over.

2.Stir in capers, parsley, and lemon zest. Shape cakes out of the mixture and dust them with flour. Refrigerate for 1 hour.

3.Preheat the air fryer to 350 F. Remove the cakes and brush them with olive oil.

4.Bake in the greased frying basket for 12-14 minutes, flipping once halfway through cooking. Serve with ketchup. Enjoy!

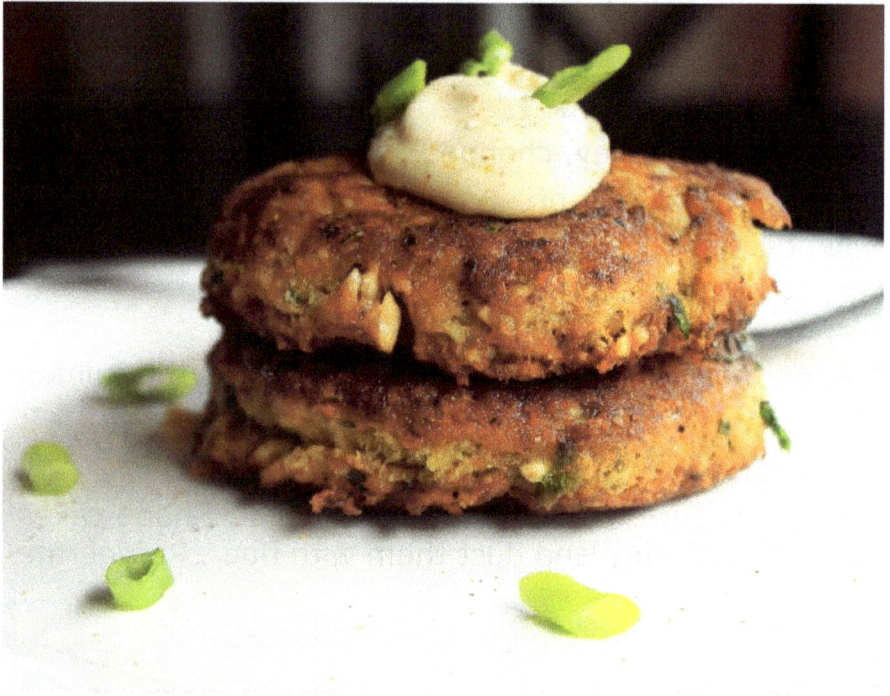

# Parmesan Tilapia Fillets

**Cooking Time:**

15 minutes

**Servings:**4

**Ingredients:**

¾ cup Parmesan cheese, grated

2 tbsp olive oil

2 tsp paprika

2 tbsp fresh parsley, chopped

¼ tsp garlic powder

4 tilapia fillets

**Directions:**

1.Preheat air fryer to 350 F. Mix parsley, Parmesan cheese, garlic, and paprika in a shallow bowl.

2.Coat fillets with the Parmesan mixture and brush with the olive oil. Place the filets into the air fryer basket and Air Fryer for 10-12 minutes, flipping once until golden brown. Serve immediately

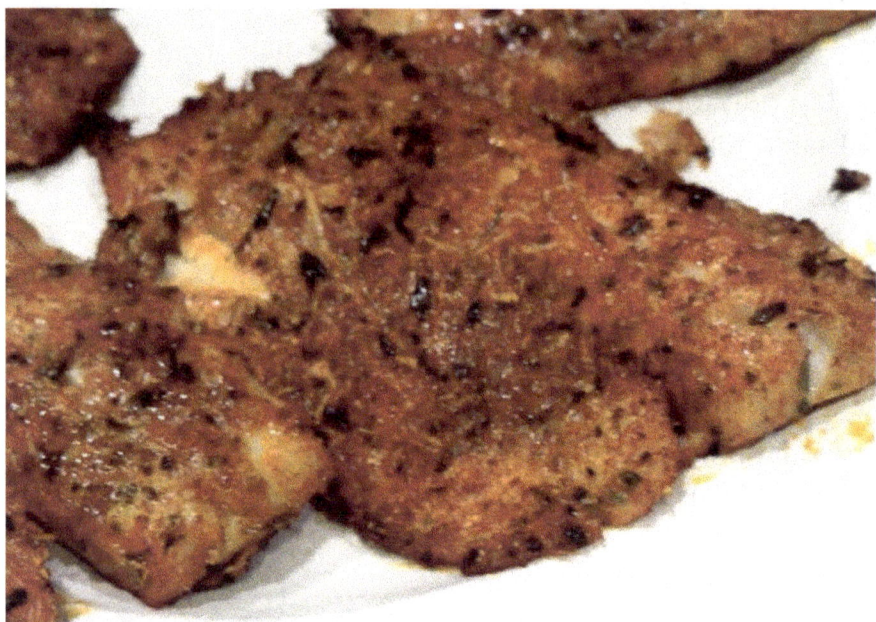

# Spicy Shrimp with Coconut-Avocado Dip

**Cooking Time:**

15 minutes

**Servings:**4

**Ingredients:**

1 ¼ lb tiger shrimp, peeled and deveined

2 garlic cloves, minced

¼ tsp red chili flakes

1 lime, juiced and zested

Salt to taste

1 tbsp fresh cilantro, chopped

1 large avocado, pitted

¼ cup coconut cream

2 tablespoons olive oil

**Directions:**

1.Blend avocado, lime juice, coconut cream, cilantro, olive oil, and salt in a food processor until smooth.

2.Transfer to a bowl, cover, and keep in the fridge until ready to use. Preheat air fryer to 390 F.

3.In a bowl, place garlic, chili flakes, lime zest, and salt, and add in the shrimp; toss to coat.

4.Place them in the frying basket and Air Fryer for 8-10 minutes, shaking once halfway through or until entirely pink. Serve with the chilled avocado dip.

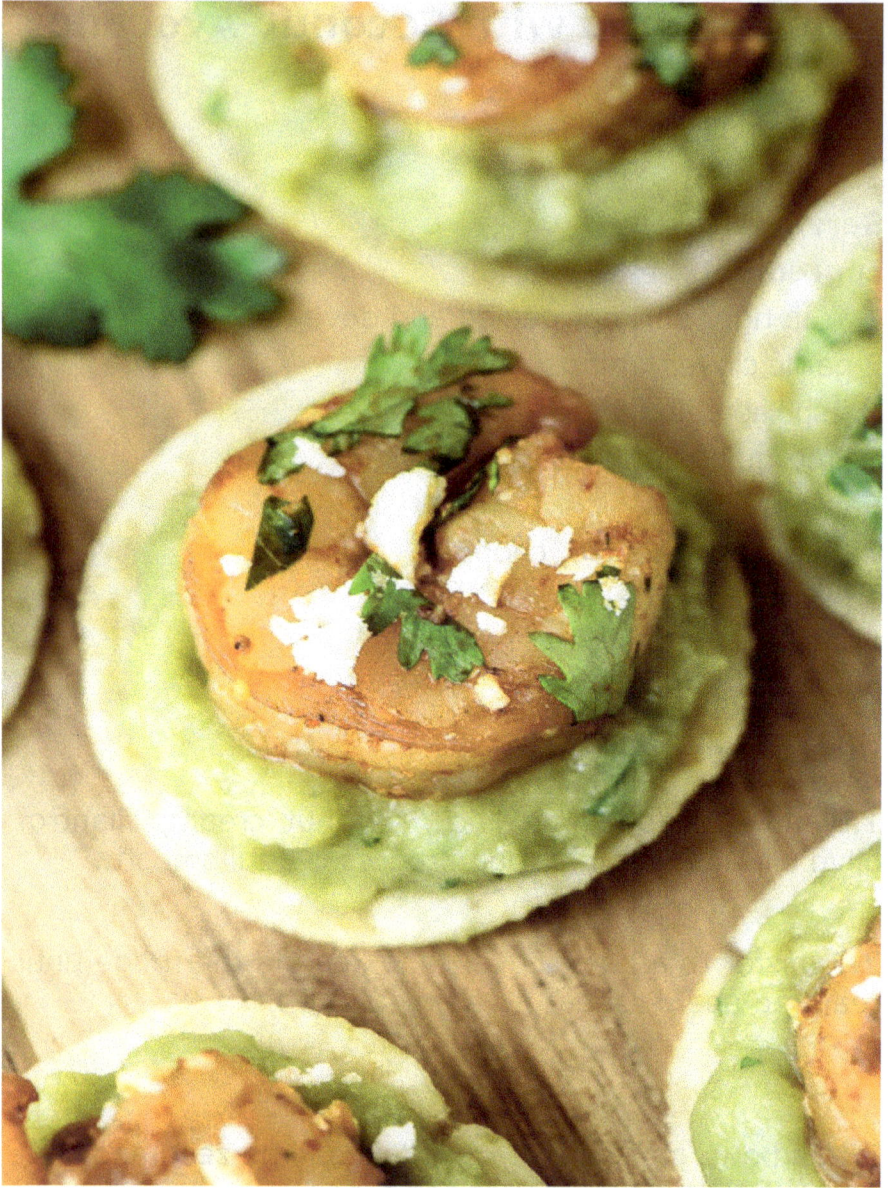

# Calamari Rings with Olives

**Cooking Time:**

30 minutes

**Servings:**4

**Ingredients:**

1 lb calamari rings

2 tbsp cilantro, chopped

1 chili pepper, minced

2 tbsp olive oil

1 cup pimiento-stuffed green olives

Salt and black pepper to taste

**Directions:**

1.In a bowl, add calamari rings, chili pepper, salt, black pepper, olive oil, and fresh cilantro. Marinate for 10 minutes.

2.Pour the calamari into a baking dish and place it inside the fryer. Air Fryer for 15 minutes, stirring every 5 minutes at 400 F. Serve warm with pimiento-stuffed olives.

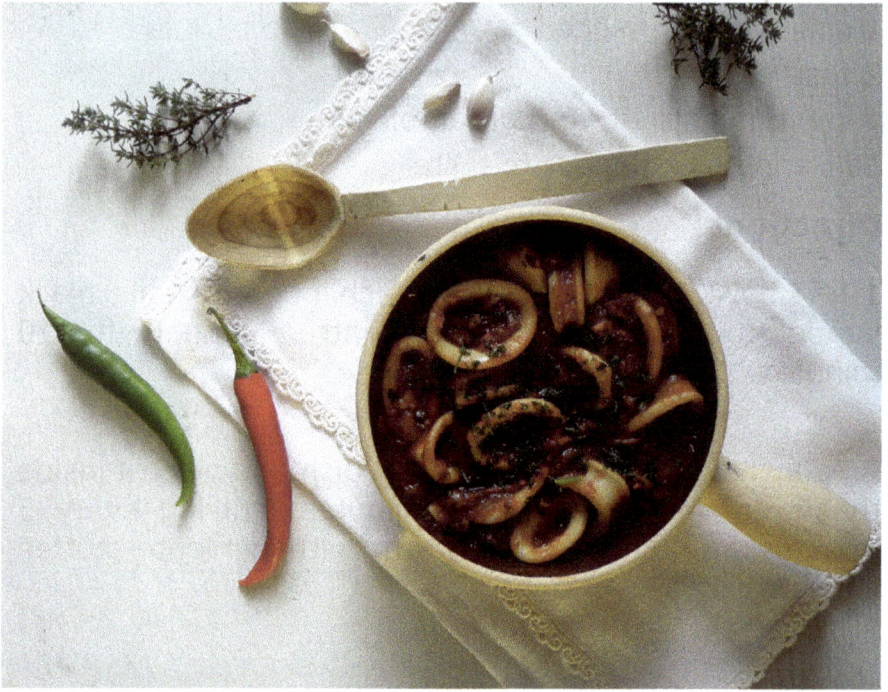

# Cajun Mango Salmon

**Cooking Time:**

15 minutes
**Servings:**4
**Ingredients:**

4 salmon fillets

½ tsp brown sugar

1 tbsp Cajun seasoning

1 lemon, zested and juiced

1 tbsp fresh parsley, chopped

2 tbsp mango salsa

**Directions:**

1.Preheat air fryer to 350 F. In a bowl, mix sugar, Cajun seasoning, lemon juice and zest, and coat the salmon with the mixture.

2.Line with parchment paper the frying basket and place in the fish. Bake for 12 minutes, turning once halfway through. Top with parsley and mango salsa to serve.

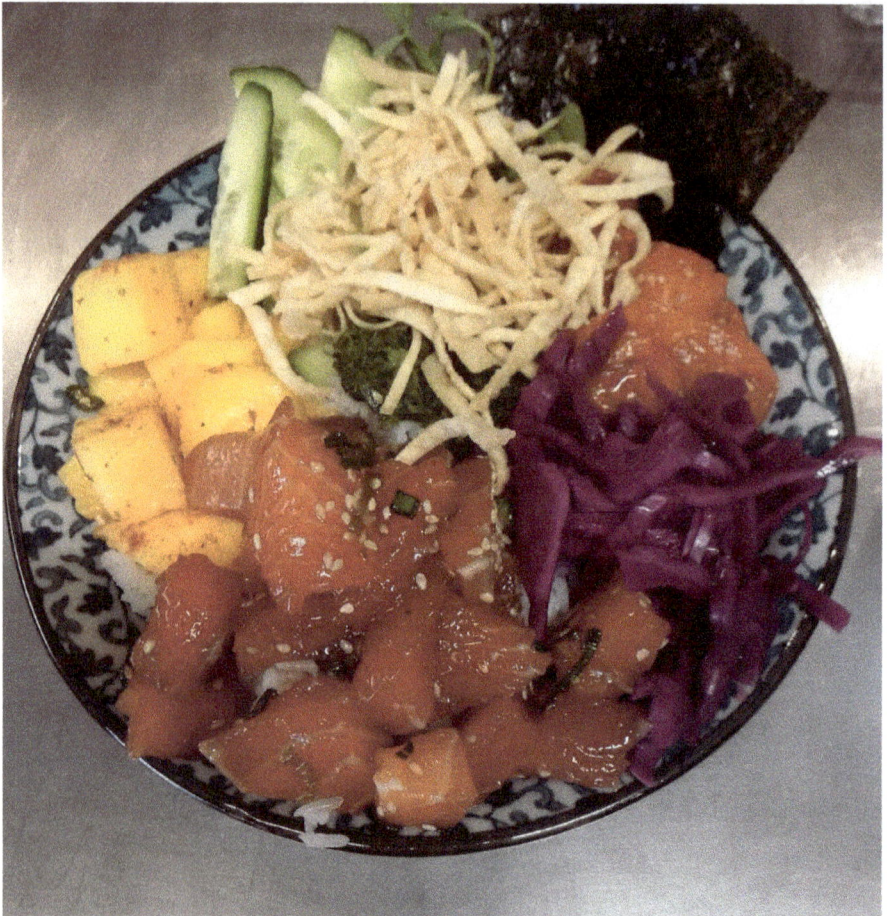

# Fried Tilapia Bites

**Cooking Time:**

20 minutes

**Servings:**4

**Ingredients:**

1 lb tilapia fillets, cut into chunks

½ cup cornflakes

1 cup flour

2 eggs, beaten

Salt to taste Lemon wedges for serving

**Directions:**

1.Preheat air fryer to 390 F. Pour the flour, eggs, and cornflakes each into different bowls. Dip the tilapia first in the flour, then in the egg, and lastly, coat with the cornflakes.

2.Lay on the greased air fryer basket and Air Fryer for 6 minutes. Shake and cook for 4-5 minutes until crispy. Serve with lemon wedges. Enjoy!

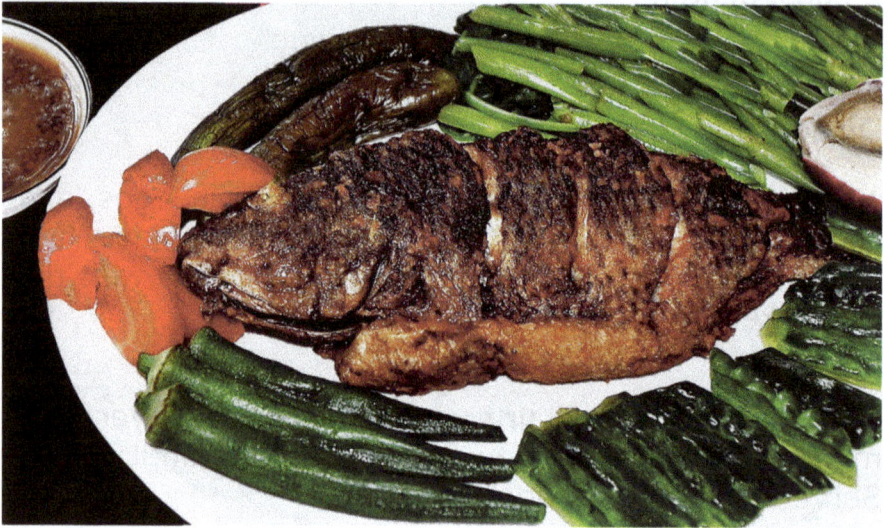

# Salmon Bowl with Lime Drizzle

**Preparation time:**

30 minutes

**Servings:**2

**Ingredients:**

1pound salmon steak

2 teaspoons sesame oil

Sea salt and Sichuan pepper, to taste

1/2 teaspoon coriander seeds

1 lime, juiced

2 tablespoons reduced-sodium soy sauce

1 teaspoon honey

**Directions:**

1.Pat the salmon dry and drizzle it with 1 teaspoon of sesame oil. Season the salmon with salt, pepper and coriander seeds.

2.Transfer the salmon to the Air Fryer cooking basket. Cook the salmon at 400 degrees F for 5 minutes; turn the salmon over and continue to cook for 5 minutes more or until opaque.

3.Meanwhile, warm the remaining ingredients in a small saucepan to make the lime drizzle.

4.Slice the fish into bite-sized strips, drizzle with the sauce and serve immediately. Enjoy!

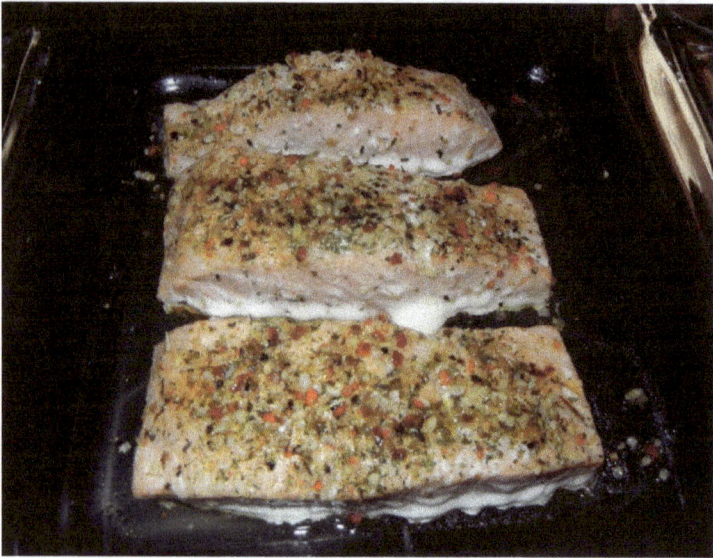

# Classic Calamari with Mediterranean Sauce

**Cooking Time:**

15 minutes

**Servings:** 2

**Ingredients:**

1/2 pound calamari tubes cut into rings, cleaned

Sea salt and ground black pepper, to season

1/2 cup almond flour

1/2 cup all-purpose flour

4 tablespoons parmesan cheese, grated

1/2 cup ale beer

1/4 teaspoon cayenne pepper

1/2 cup breadcrumbs

1/4 cup mayonnaise

1/4 cup Greek-style yogurt

1 clove garlic, minced

1 tablespoon fresh lemon juice

1 teaspoon fresh parsley, chopped

1 teaspoon fresh dill, chopped

**Directions:**

1. Sprinkle the calamari with salt and black pepper. Mix the flour, cheese and beer in a bowl until well combined.
2.

2. In another bowl, mix cayenne pepper and breadcrumbs.00Dip the calamari pieces in the flour mixture, then roll them onto the breadcrumb mixture, pressing to coat on all sides; transfer them to a lightly oiled cooking basket.

3.Cook at 400 degrees F for 4 minutes, shaking the basket halfway through the cooking time.

4.Meanwhile, mix the remaining ingredients until everything is well incorporated. Serve warm calamari with the sauce for dipping. Enjoy!

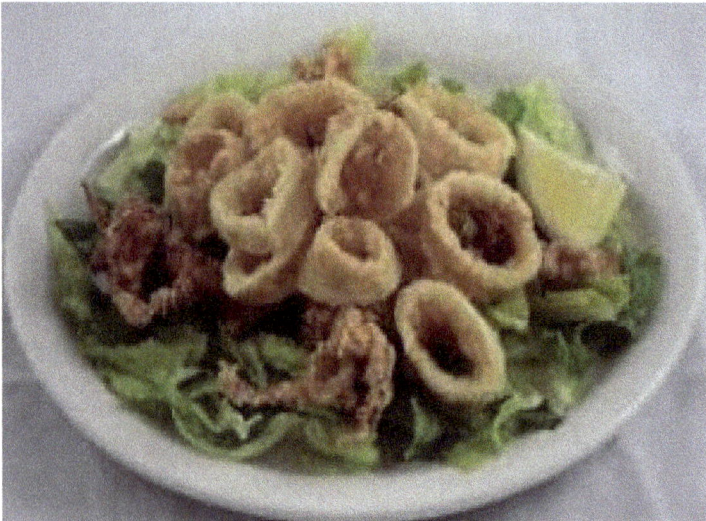

# Herb and Garlic Grouper Filets

**Cooking Time:**

15 minutes

**Servings:** 3

**Ingredients:**

1pound grouper filets

1/4 teaspoon shallot powder

1/4 teaspoon porcini powder

1 teaspoon fresh garlic, minced

1/2 teaspoon cayenne pepper

1/2 teaspoon hot paprika

1/4 teaspoon oregano

1/2 teaspoon marjoram

1/2 teaspoon sage

1 tablespoon butter, melted

Sea salt and black pepper, to taste

**Directions:**

1.Pat dry the grouper filets using kitchen towels. In a small dish, make the rub by mixing the remaining ingredients until everything is well incorporated.

2.Rub the fish with the mixture, coating well on all sides. Cook the grouper filets in the preheated Air Fryer at 400 degrees F for 5 minutes; turn the filets over and cook on the other side for 5 minutes more. Serve over hot rice if desired. Enjoy!

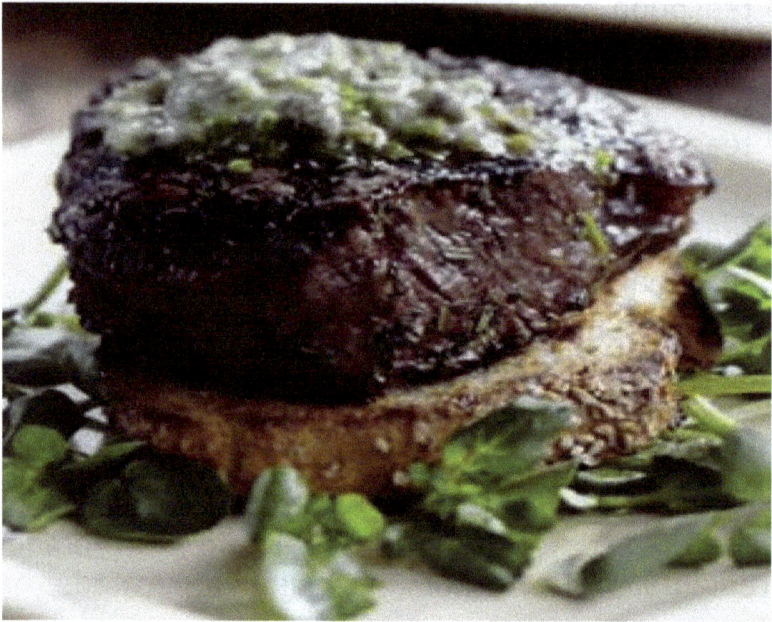

# Crab Cake Burgers

**Cook Time:**

2hours   20

**Servings:**3

**INGREDIE**

**NT**

1eggs, beaten
1 shallot, chopped
2 garlic cloves, crushed
1 tablespoon olive oil
1 teaspoon yellow mustard
1 teaspoon fresh cilantro, chopped
10 ounces crab meat
1 cup tortilla chips, crushed
1/2 teaspoon cayenne pepper
1/2 teaspoon ground black pepper
Sea salt, to taste
3/4 cup fresh bread crumbs

**Directions:**

1.In a mixing bowl, thoroughly combine the eggs, shallot, garlic, olive oil, mustard, cilantro, crab meat, tortilla chips, cayenne pepper, black pepper, and salt. Mix until well combined.

2.Shape the mixture into 6 patties. Dip the crab patties into the fresh breadcrumbs, coating well on all sides. Place in your refrigerator for 2 hours.

3.Spritz the crab patties with cooking oil on both sides. Cook in the preheated Air Fryer at 360 degrees F for 14 minutes. Serve on dinner rolls if desired. Enjoy!

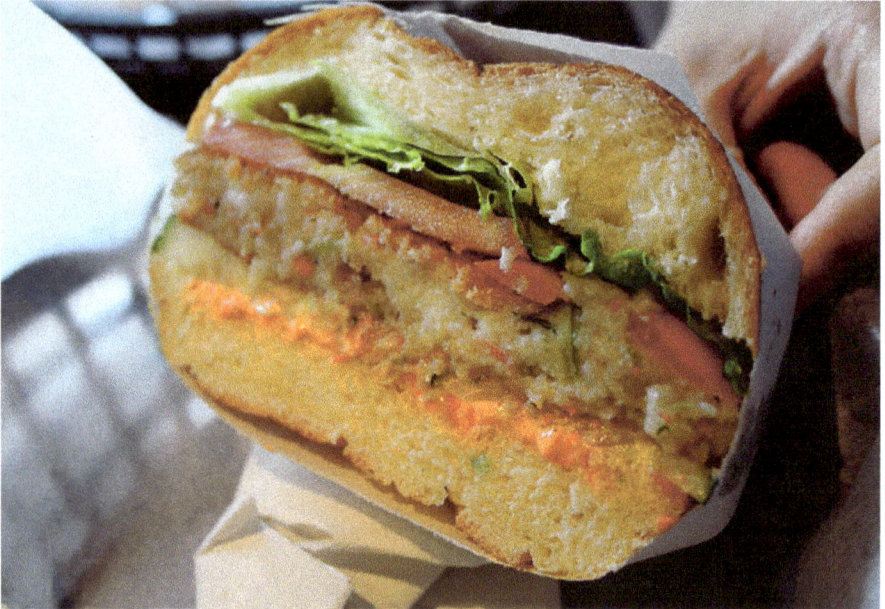

# Cajun Cod Fillets with Avocado Sauce

**Cooking Time:**

20 minutes

**Servings:** 2

**Ingredients:**

2 cod fish fillets

1 egg

Sea salt, to taste

1/2 cup tortilla chips, crushed

2 teaspoons olive oil

1/2 avocado, peeled, pitted, and mashed

1 tablespoon mayonnaise

3 tablespoons sour cream

1/2 teaspoon yellow mustard

1 teaspoon lemon juice

1 garlic clove, minced

1⊠ teaspoon black pepper

1⊠ teaspoon salt

1⊠ teaspoon hot pepper sauce

## Directions:

1.Start by preheating your Air Fryer to 360 degrees F. Spritz the Air Fryer basket with cooking oil.

2.Pat dry the fish fillets with a kitchen towel. Beat the egg in a shallow bowl. In a separate bowl, thoroughly combine the salt, crushed tortilla chips, and olive oil.

3.Dip the fish into the egg, then, into the crumb mixture, making sure to coat thoroughly.

4.Cook in the preheated Air Fryer approximately 12 minutes. Meanwhile, make the avocado sauce by mixing the remaining ingredients in a bowl.

4.Place in your refrigerator until ready to serve. Serve the fish fillets with chilled avocado sauce on the side. Enjoy!

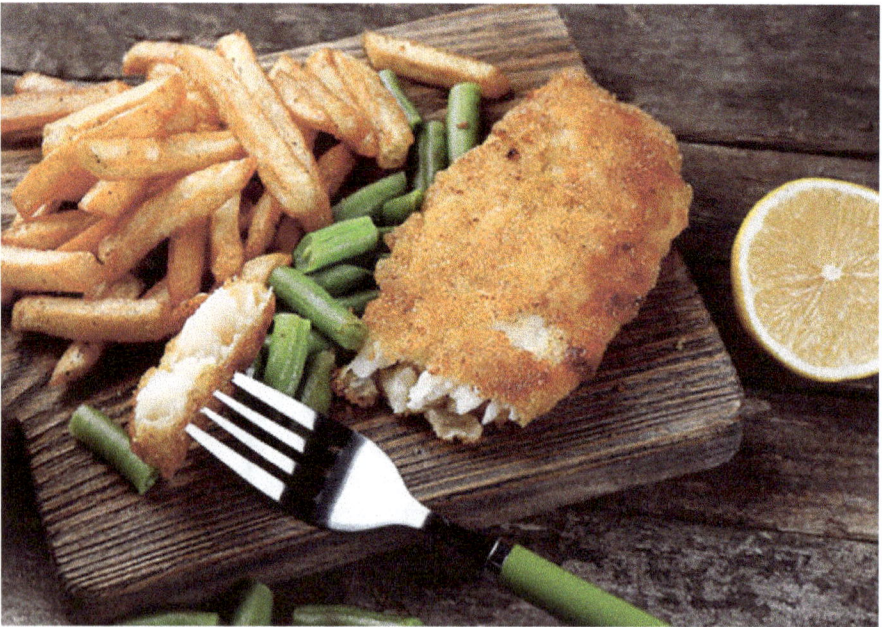

# Snapper Casserole with Gruyere Cheese

## Cooking Time:

25 minutes

**Servings:**4

**Ingredients:**

2 tablespoons olive oil

1 shallot, thinly sliced

2 garlic cloves, minced

1 ½ pounds snapper fillets

Sea salt and ground black pepper, to taste

1 teaspoon cayenne pepper

1/2 teaspoon dried basil

1/2 cup tomato puree

1/2 cup white wine

1 cup Gruyere cheese, shredded

## Directions:

1.Heat 1 tablespoon of olive oil in a saucepan over medium-high heat. Now, cook the shallot and garlic until tender and aromatic.

2.Preheat your Air Fryer to 370 degrees F. Grease a casserole dish with 1 tablespoon of olive oil.

3.Place the snapper fillet in the casserole dish. Season with salt, black pepper, and cayenne pepper. Add the sautéed shallot mixture.

4.Add the basil, tomato puree and wine to the casserole dish. Cook for 10 minutes in the preheated Air Fryer. Top with the shredded cheese and cook an additional 7 minutes. Serve immediately

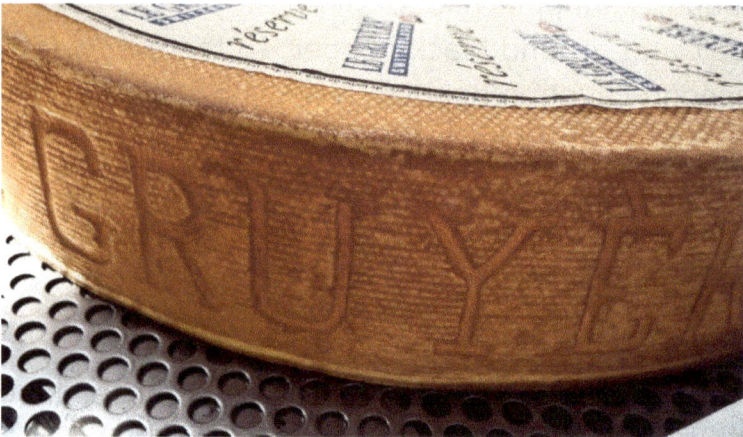

# Halibut with Thai Lemongrass Marinade

**Cooking Time:**

45 minutes

**Servings:**2

**Ingredients:**

2 tablespoons tamari sauce

2 tablespoons fresh lime juice

2 tablespoons olive oil

1 teaspoon Thai curry paste

1/2 inch lemongrass, finely chopped

1 teaspoon basil

2 cloves garlic, minced

2 tablespoons shallot, minced

Sea salt and ground black pepper, to taste

2 halibut steaks

**Directions:**

1.Place all ingredients in a ceramic dish; let it marinate for 30 minutes. Place the halibut steaks in the lightly greased cooking basket.

2.Bake in the preheated Air Fryer at 400 degrees F for 9 to 10 minutes, basting with the reserved marinade and flipping them halfway through the cooking time. Enjoy!

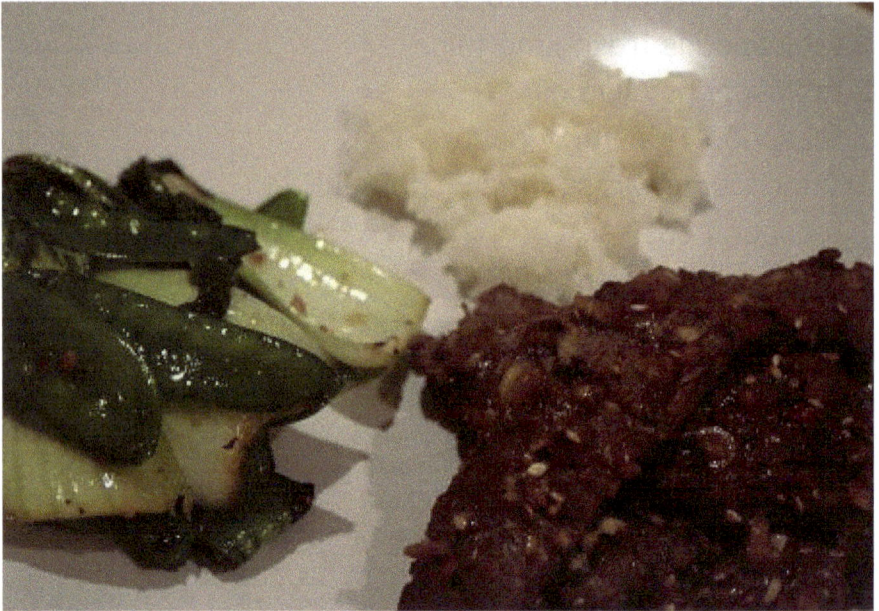

# Tuna Cake Burgers with Beer Cheese Sauce

**Cook Time:**

2hours    20

**minutes**

**Servings:**4

**INGREDIE**

**NT**

pound canned tuna, drained
1 egg, whisked
1 garlic clove, minced
2 tablespoons shallots, minced
1 cup fresh breadcrumbs
Sea salt and ground black pepper, to taste
1 tablespoon sesame oil

Beer Cheese Sauce:

1 tablespoon butter

1 cup beer

1 tablespoon rice flour

2 tablespoons Colby cheese, grated

**Directions:**

1.In a mixing bowl, thoroughly combine the tuna, egg, garlic, shallots, breadcrumbs, salt, and black pepper.

2.Shape the tuna mixture into four patties and place in your refrigerator for 2 hours. Brush the patties with sesame oil on both sides.

3.Cook in the preheated Air Fryer at 360 degrees F for 14 minutes. In the meantime, melt the butter in a pan over a moderate heat.

4.Add the beer and flour and whisk until it starts bubbling.

5.Now, stir in the grated cheese and cook for 3 to 4 minutes longer or until the cheese has melted. Spoon the sauce over the fish cake burgers and serve immediately.

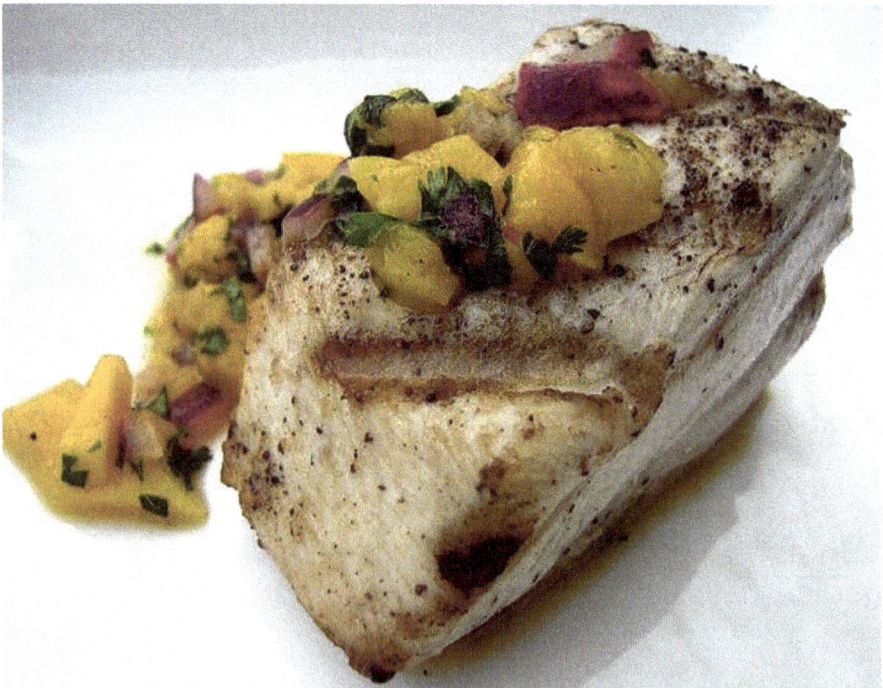

# Easiest Lobster Tails Ever

**Cooking Time:**

25 minutes

**Servings:2**

**Ingredients:**

6-ounce lobster tails

1 teaspoon fresh cilantro, minced

1/2 teaspoon dried rosemary

1/2 teaspoon garlic, pressed

1 teaspoon deli mustard

Sea salt and ground black pepper, to taste

1 teaspoon olive oil

**Directions:**

1.Toss the lobster tails with the other ingredients until they are well coated on all sides. Cook the lobster tails at 370 degrees F for 3 minutes.

2.Then, turn them and cook on the other side for 3 to 4 minutes more until they are opaque. Serve warm and enjoy!

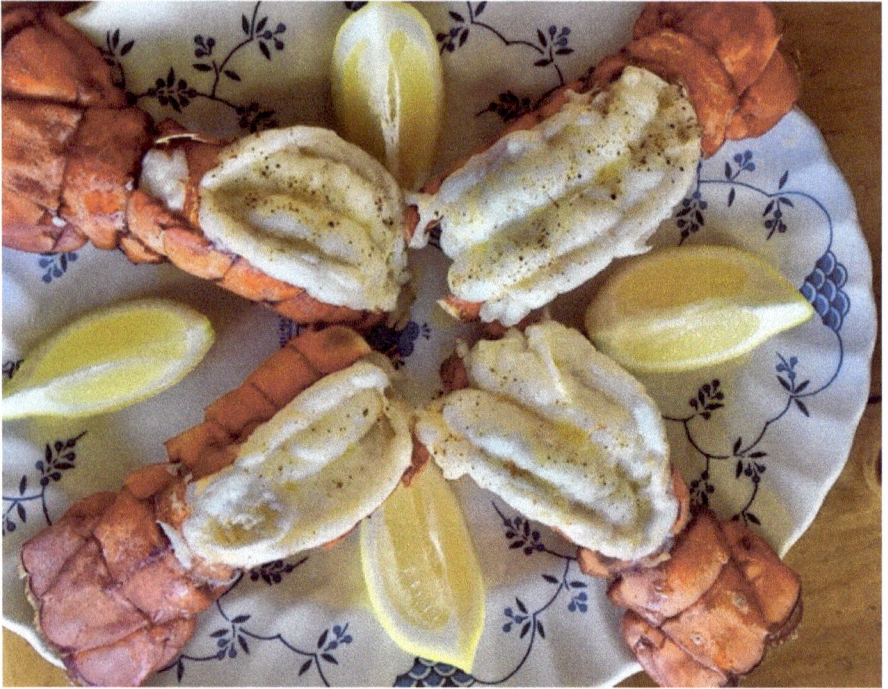

# Grouper with Miso-Honey Sauce

**Cooking Time:**

15 minutes

**Servings:**2

**Ingredients:**

3/4 pound grouper fillets

Salt and white pepper, to taste

1 tablespoon sesame oil

1 teaspoon water

1 teaspoon deli mustard or Dijon mustard

1/4 cup white miso

1 tablespoon mirin

1 tablespoon honey

1 tablespoon Shoyu sauce

**Directions:**

1.Sprinkle the grouper fillets with salt and white pepper; drizzle them with a nonstick cooking oil. Cook the fish at 400 degrees F for 5 minutes; turn the fish fillets over and cook an additional 5 minutes.

2.Meanwhile, make the sauce by whisking the remaining ingredients.

3.Serve the warm fish with the miso-honey sauce on the side.

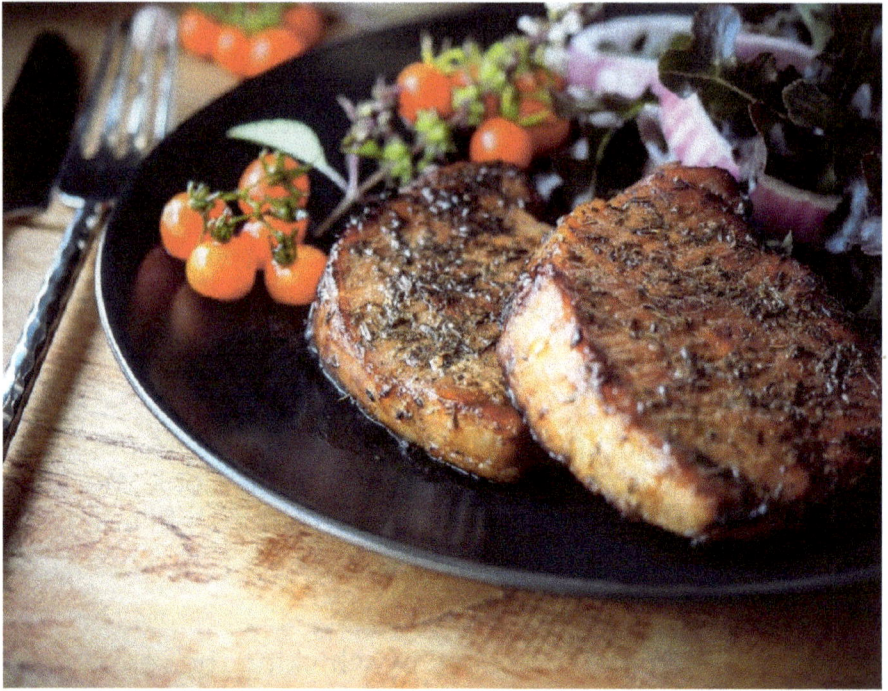

# Southwestern Prawns with Asparagus

**Cooking Time:**

10 minutes

**Servings:** 3

**Ingredients:**

1pound prawns, deveined

1/2pound asparagus spears, cut into1-inch chinks

1 teaspoon butter, melted

1/4 teaspoon oregano

1/2 teaspoon mixed peppercorns, crushed

Salt, to taste

1 ripe avocado

1 lemon, sliced

1/2 cup chunky-style salsa

## *Directions:*

1.Toss your prawns and asparagus with melted butter, oregano, salt and mixed peppercorns.

2.Cook the prawns and asparagus at 400 degrees F for 5 minutes, shaking the basket halfway through the cooking time.

3.Divide the prawns and asparagus between serving plates and garnish with avocado and lemon slices. Serve with the salsa on the side. Enjoy!

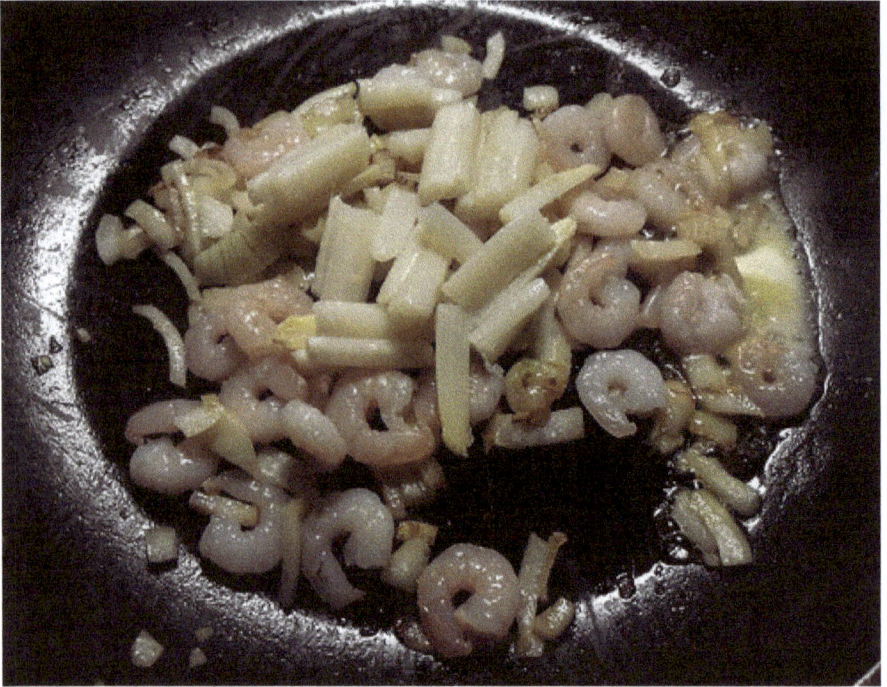

# Homemade Fish Fingers

**Cooking Time:**

15 minutes

**Servings:** 2

**Ingredients:**

3/4 pound tilapia

1 egg

2 tablespoons milk

4 tablespoons chickpea flour

1/4 cup pork rinds

1/2 cup breadcrumbs

1/2 teaspoon red chili flakes

Coarse sea salt and black pepper, to season

**Directions:**

1.Rinse the tilapia and pat it dry using kitchen towels. Then, cut the tilapia into strips.

2.Then, whisk the egg, milk and chickpea flour in a rimmed plate. Add the pork rinds and breadcrumbs to another plate; stir in red chili flakes, salt and black pepper and stir to combine well.

3.Dip the fish strips in the egg mixture, then, roll them over the breadcrumb mixture. Transfer the fish fingers to the Air Fryer cooking basket and spritz them with a nonstick cooking spray.

4.Cook in the preheated Air Fryer at 400 degrees F for 10 minutes, shaking the basket halfway through to ensure even browning. Serve warm and enjoy.

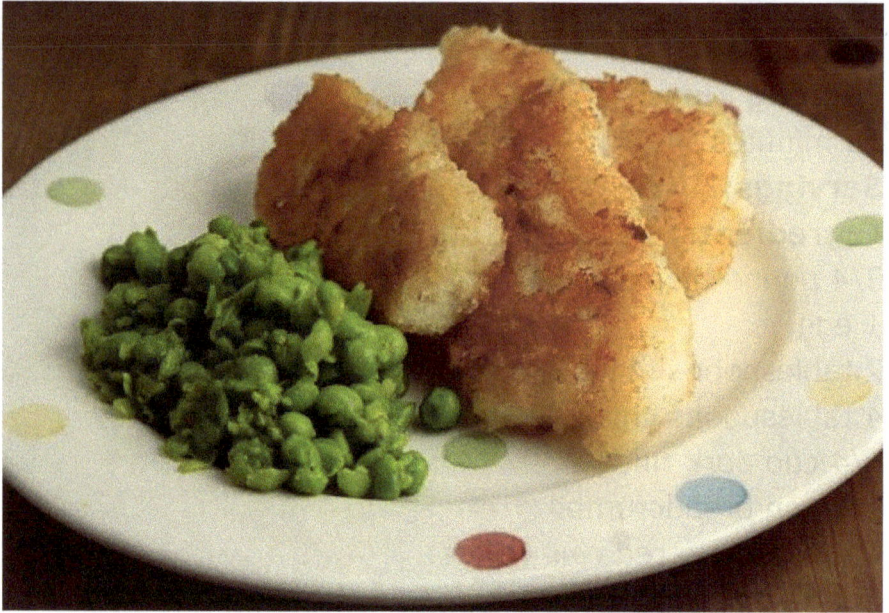

# Dijon Catfish with Eggplant Sauce

**Cooking Time:**

30 minutes

**Servings**:3

**Ingredients:**

1 pound catfish fillets

Sea salt and ground black pepper, to taste

1/4 cup Dijon mustard
1 tablespoon honey
1 tablespoon white vinegar
1 pound eggplant,
1 ½-inch cubes
2 tablespoons olive oil
1 tablespoon tahini
1/2 teaspoon garlic, minced
1 tablespoon parsley, chopped

**Directions:**

1.Pat the catfish dry with paper towels and generously season with salt and black pepper.


2.In a small mixing bowl, thoroughly combine Dijon mustard, honey and vinegar. Cook the fish in your Air Fryer at 400 degrees F for 5 minutes.


3.Turn the fish over and brush with the Dijon mixture; continue to cook for a further 5 minutes. Then, set your Air Fryer to 400 degrees F.

4.Add the eggplant chunks to the cooking basket and cook for 15 minutes, shaking the basket occasionally to ensure even cooking.

5.Transfer the cooked eggplant to a bowl of your food processor; stir in the remaining ingredients and blitz until everything is well blended and smooth. Serve the warm catfish with the eggplant sauce on the side.

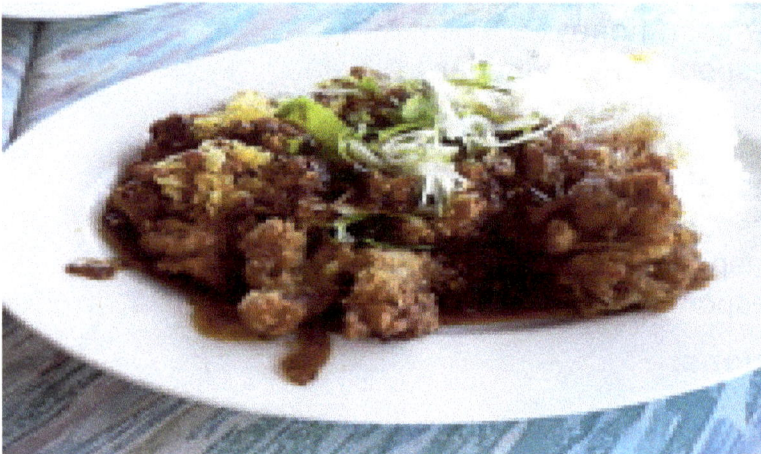

# Scallops with Pineapple Salsa and Pickled Onions

**Cooking Time:**

15 minutes

**Servings:**4

**Ingredients:**

12 scallops

1 teaspoon sesame oil

1/4 teaspoon dried rosemary

1/2 teaspoon dried tarragon

1/2 teaspoon dried basil

1/4 teaspoon red pepper flakes, crushed

Coarse sea salt and black pepper, to taste

1/2 cup pickled onions, drained

Pineapple Salsa:

1 cup pineapple, diced

2 tablespoons fresh cilantro, roughly chopped

1 jalapeño, deveined and minced

1 small-sized red onion, minced

1 teaspoon ginger root, peeled and grated

1/2 teaspoon coconut sugar

Sea salt and ground black pepper, to taste

## Directions:

1.Toss the scallops sesame oil, rosemary, tarragon, basil, red pepper, salt and black pepper.

3.Cook in the preheated Air Fryer at 400 degrees F for 6 to 7 minutes, shaking the basket once or twice to ensure even cooking.

4.Meanwhile, process all the salsa ingredients in your blender; cover and place the salsa in your refrigerator until ready to serve. Serve the warm scallops with pickled onions and pineapple salsa on the side. Enjoy!

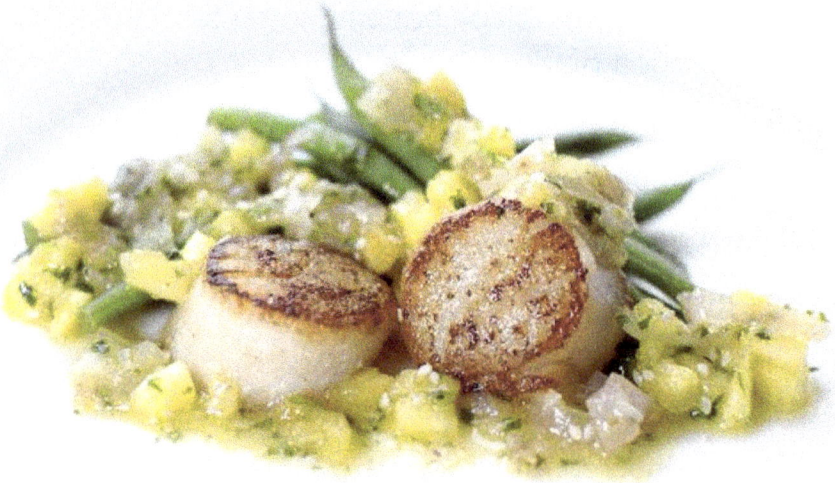

# Korean-Style Salmon Patties

**Cooking Time:**

15 minutes

**Servings:**4

**Ingredients:**

1pound salmon

1 egg

1 garlic clove, minced

2 green onions, minced

1/2 cup rolled oats

## Sauce:

1 teaspoon rice wine

1 ½ tablespoons soy sauce

1 teaspoon honey

A pinch of salt

1 teaspoon gochugaru Korean red chili pepper flakes

## Directions:

1.Start by preheating your Air Fryer to 380 degrees F. Spritz the Air Fryer basket with cooking oil.

2.Mix the salmon, egg, garlic, green onions, and rolled oats in a bowl; knead with your hands until everything is well incorporated.

3.Shape the mixture into equally sized patties. Transfer your patties to the Air Fryer basket. Cook the fish patties for 10 minutes, turning them over halfway through.

4.Meanwhile, make the sauce by whisking all ingredients. Serve the warm fish patties with the sauce on the side. Enjoy!

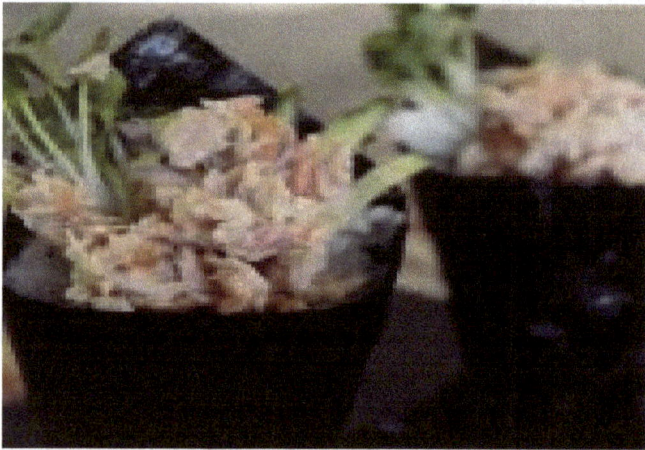

# Halibut Cakes with Horseradish Mayo

**Cooking Time:**

20 minutes

**Servings:**4

**Ingredients:**

**Halibut Cakes:**

1 pound halibut

2 tablespoons olive oil

1/2 teaspoon cayenne pepper

1/4 teaspoon black pepper

Salt, to taste

2 tablespoons cilantro, chopped

1 shallot, chopped

2 garlic cloves, minced

1/2 cup Romano cheese, grated

1/2 cup breadcrumbs

1 egg, whisked

1 tablespoon Worcestershire sauce

Mayo Sauce:

1 teaspoon horseradish, grated

1/2 cup mayonnaise

**Directions:**

1.Start by preheating your Air Fryer to 380 degrees F. Spritz the Air Fryer basket with cooking oil.

2.Mix all ingredients for the halibut cakes in a bowl; knead with your hands until everything is well incorporated.

3.Shape the mixture into equally sized patties. Transfer your patties to the Air Fryer basket.

4.Cook the fish patties for 10 minutes, turning them over halfway through. Mix the horseradish and mayonnaise. Serve the halibut cakes with the horseradish mayo.

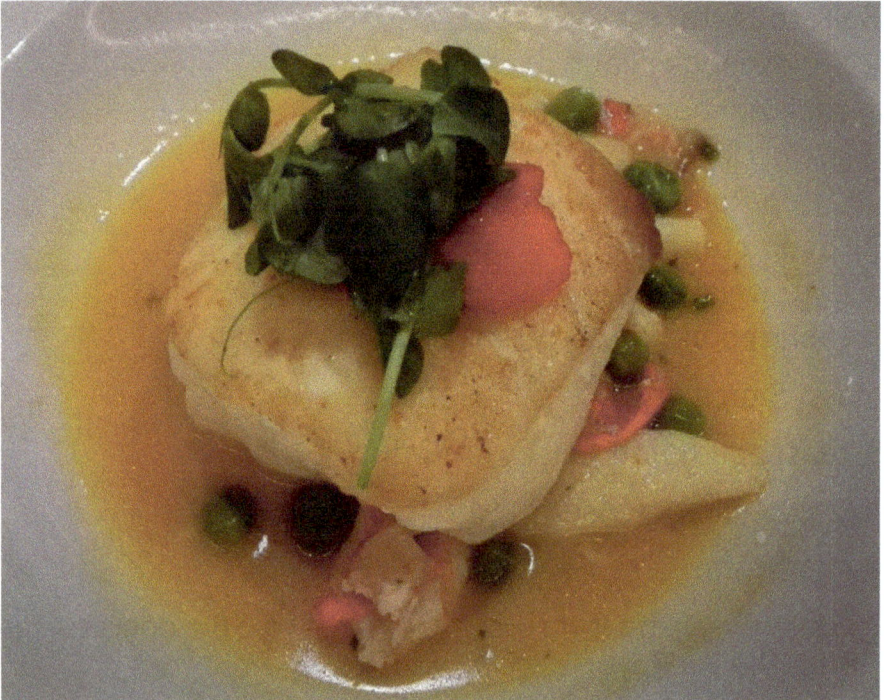

# Sunday Fish with Sticky Sauce

**Cooking Time:**
**20minutes**
**Servings:2**
**Ingredients:**

1pollack fillets

Salt and black pepper, to taste

1 tablespoon olive oil

1 cup chicken broth

2 tablespoons light soy sauce

1 tablespoon brown sugar

2 tablespoons butter, melted

1 teaspoon fresh ginger, minced

1 teaspoon fresh garlic, minced

2 corn tortillas

## Directions:

1.Pat dry the pollack fillets and season them with salt and black pepper; drizzle the sesame oil all over the fish fillets.


2.Preheat the Air Fryer to 380 degrees F and cook your fish for 11 minutes.


3.Slice into bite-sized pieces. Meanwhile, prepare the sauce. Add the broth to a large saucepan and bring to a boil.

4.Add the soy sauce, sugar, butter, ginger, and garlic. Reduce the heat to simmer and cook until it is reduced slightly.

5.Add the fish pieces to the warm sauce. Serve on corn tortillas and enjoy!

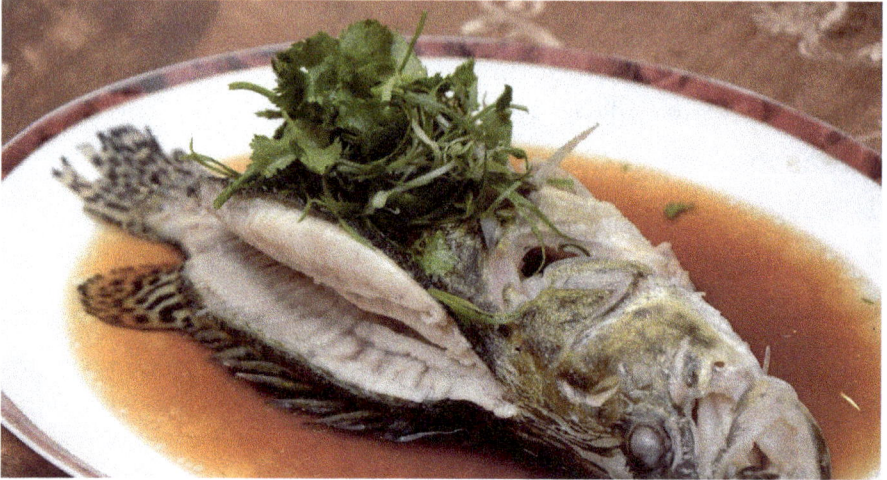

# Crusty Catfish with Sweet Potato Fries

**Cook Time:**

50   minutes

**Servings:** 2

**Ingredients:**

1/2 pound catfish

1/2 cup bran cereal

1/4 cup parmesan cheese, grated

Sea salt and ground black pepper, to taste

1 teaspoon smoked paprika

1 teaspoon garlic powder

1/4 teaspoon ground bay leaf

1 egg

2 tablespoons butter, melted

4 sweet potatoes, cut French fries

**Directions:**

1. Pat the catfish dry with a kitchen towel. Combine the bran cereal with the parmesan cheese and all spices in a shallow bowl.

2. Whisk the egg in another shallow bowl. Dip the fish in the egg mixture and turn to coat evenly; then, dredge in the bran cereal mixture, turning a couple of times to coat evenly.

3.Spritz the Air Fryer basket with cooking spray. Cook the catfish in the preheated Air Fryer at 390 degrees F for 10 minutes; turn them over and cook for 4 minutes more.

4.Then, drizzle the melted butter all over the sweet potatoes; cook them in the preheated Air Fryer at 380 degrees F for 30 minutes, shaking occasionally. Serve over the warm fish fillets. Enjoy!

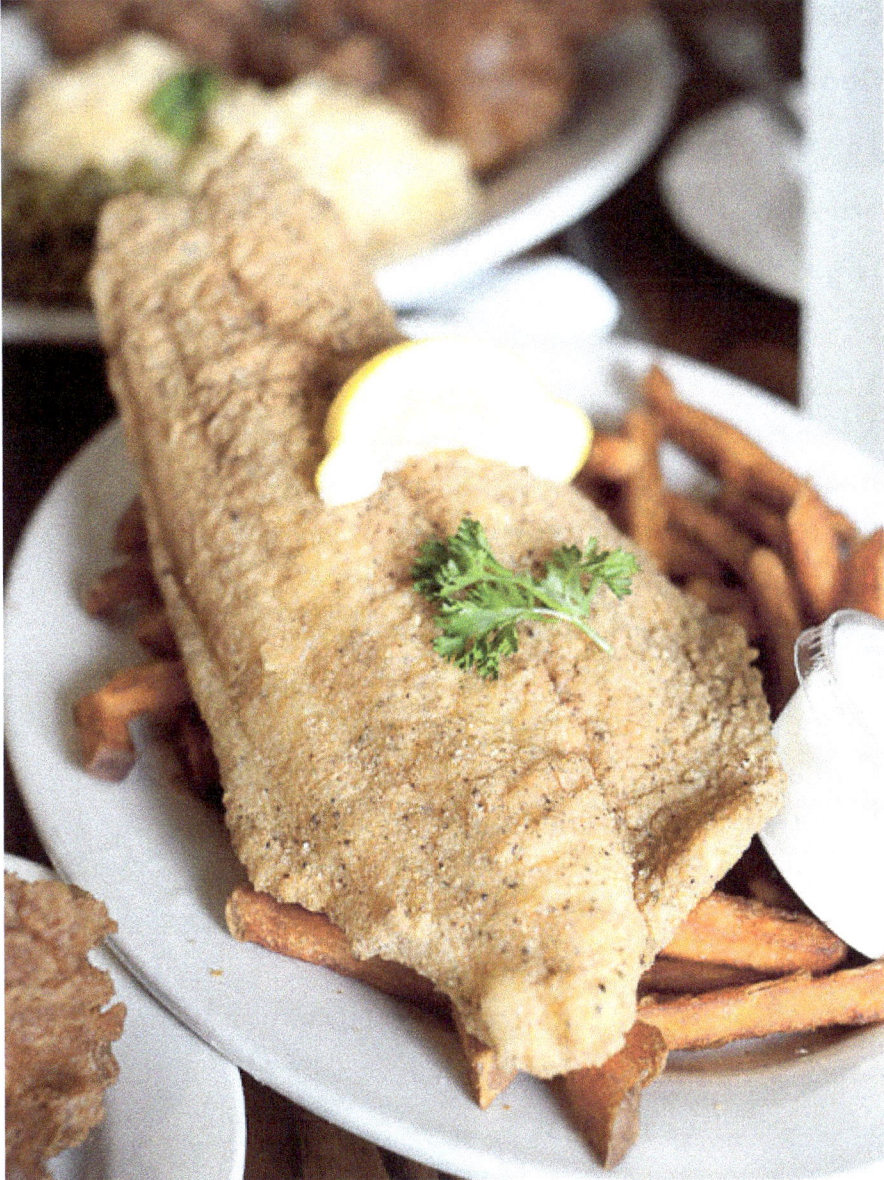

# Easy Creamy Shrimp Nachos

**Cook Time:**

15 minutes

**Servings:**4

**Ingredients:**

1pound shrimp, cleaned and deveined
1 tablespoon olive oil
2 tablespoons fresh lemon juice
1 teaspoon paprika
1/4 teaspoon cumin powder
1/2 teaspoon shallot powder
1/2 teaspoon garlic powder
Coarse sea salt and ground black pepper, to taste
1 9-ounce bag corn tortilla chips
1/4 cup pickled jalapeño, minced
1 cup Pepper Jack cheese, grated
1/2 cup sour cream

**Directions:**

1.Toss the shrimp with the olive oil, lemon juice, paprika, cumin powder, shallot powder, garlic powder, salt, and black pepper.

2.Cook in the preheated Air Fryer at 390 degrees F for 5 minutes.

3.Place the tortilla chips on the aluminum foil-lined cooking basket.

4.Top with the shrimp mixture, jalapeño and cheese. Cook another 2 minutes or until cheese has melted. Serve garnished with sour cream and enjoy!

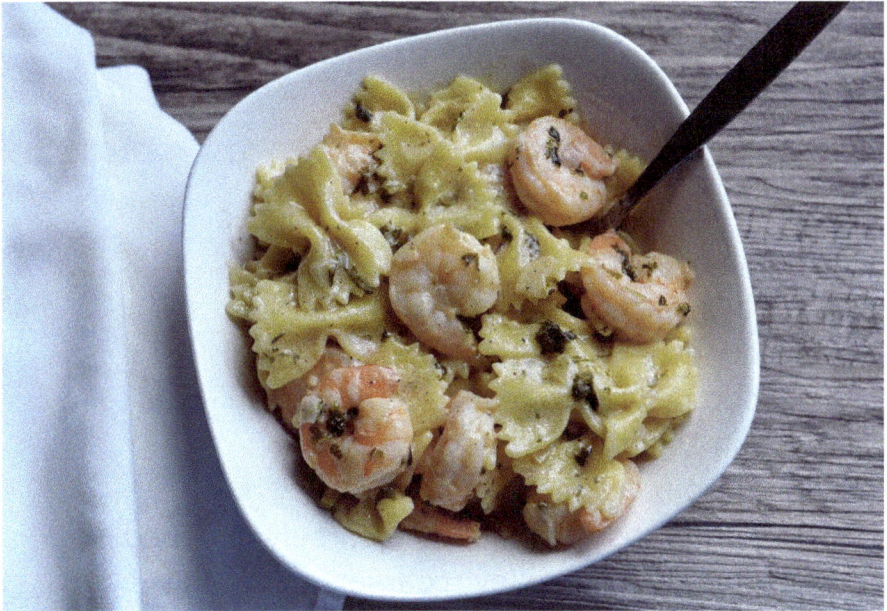

# Famous Tuna Niçoise Salad

**Cooking Time:**

15 minutes

**Servings:**4

**Ingredients:**

1 pound tuna steak

Sea salt and ground black pepper, to taste

1/2 teaspoon red pepper flakes, crushed

1/4 teaspoon dried dill weed

1/2 teaspoon garlic paste

1pound green beans, trimmed

2 handfuls baby spinach

2 handfuls iceberg lettuce, torn into pieces

1/2 red onion, sliced

1 cucumber, sliced

2 tablespoons lemon juice

1 tablespoon olive oil

1 teaspoon Dijon mustard

1 tablespoon balsamic vinegar

1 tablespoon roasted almonds, coarsely chopped

1 tablespoon fresh parsley, coarsely chopped

**Directions:**

1.Pat the tuna steak dry; toss your tuna with salt, black pepper, red pepper, dill and garlic paste. Spritz your tuna with a nonstick cooking spray.

2.Cook the tuna steak at 400 degrees F for 5 minutes; turn your tuna steak over and continue to cook for 4 to 5 minutes more.

3.Then, add the green beans to the cooking basket. Spritz green beans with a nonstick cooking spray. Cook at 400 degrees F for 5 minutes, shaking the basket once or twice.

4.Cut your tuna into thin strips and transfer to a salad bowl; add in the green beans. Then, add in the baby spinach, iceberg lettuce, onion and cucumber and toss to combine.

5.In a mixing bowl, whisk the lemon juice, olive oil, mustard and vinegar. Dress the salad and garnish with roasted almonds and fresh parsley. Serve and enjoy!

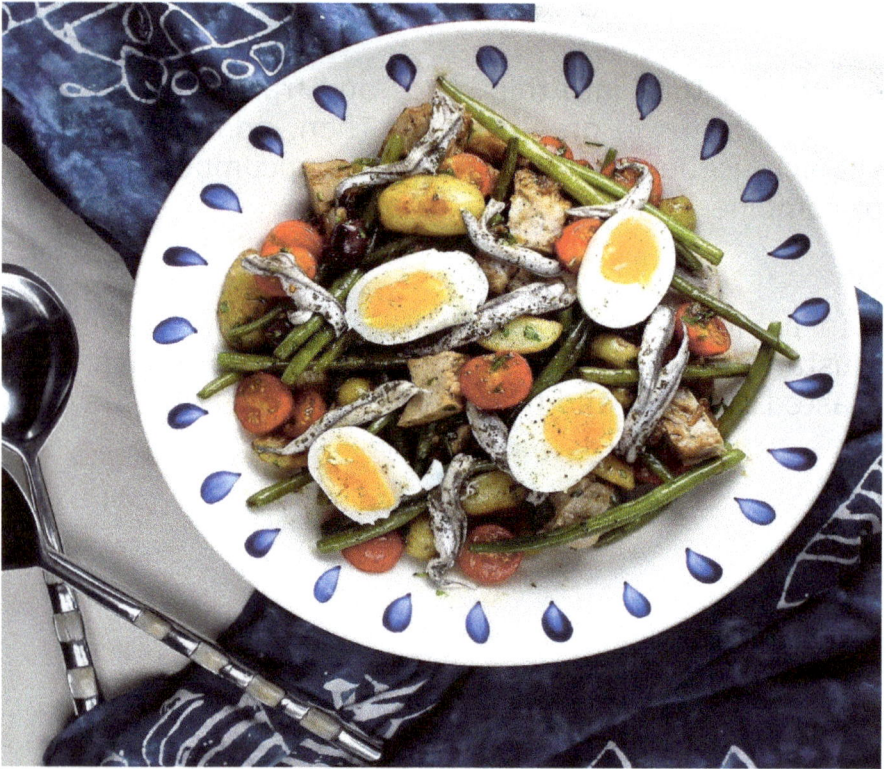

# Classic Pancetta-Wrapped Scallops

**Cook Time:**

10 minutes

**Servings:**3

**Ingredients:**

1 pound sea scallops

1 tablespoon deli mustard

2 tablespoons soy sauce

1/4 teaspoon shallot powder

1/4 teaspoon garlic powder

1/2 teaspoon dried dill

Sea salt and ground black pepper, to taste

4 ounces pancetta slices

**Directions:**

Pat dry the sea scallops and transfer them to a mixing bowl. Toss the sea scallops with the deli mustard, soy sauce, shallot powder, garlic powder, dill, salt and black pepper.


2.Wrap a slice of bacon around each scallop and transfer them to the Air Fryer cooking basket.


3.Cook in your Air Fryer at 400 degrees F for 4 minutes; turn them over and cook an additional 3 minutes. Serve with hot sauce for dipping if desired. Enjoy!

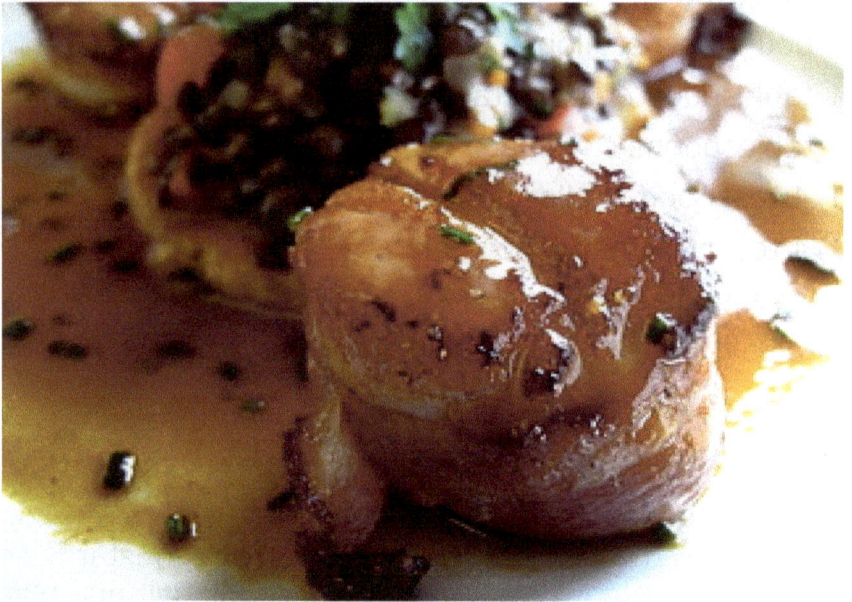

# Fried Oysters with Kaffir Lime Sauce

**Cooking Time:**

10 minutes

**Servings:** 2

**Ingredients:**

8 fresh oysters, shucked

1/3 cup plain flour

1 egg

3/4 cup breadcrumbs

1/2 teaspoon Italian seasoning mix

1 lime, freshly squeezed

1 teaspoon coconut sugar

1 kaffir lime leaf, shredded

1 habanero pepper, minced

1 teaspoon olive oil

**Directions:**

1.Clean the oysters and set them aside. Add the flour to a rimmed plate.

2.Whisk the egg in another rimmed plate. Mix the breadcrumbs and Italian seasoning mix in a third plate.

3.Dip your oysters in the flour, shaking off the excess. Then, dip them in the egg mixture and finally, coat your oysters with the breadcrumb mixture.

4.Spritz the breaded oysters with a nonstick cooking spray. Cook your oysters in the preheated Air Fryer at 400 degrees F for 2 to 3 minutes, shaking the basket halfway through the cooking time.

5.Meanwhile, blend the remaining ingredients to make the sauce. Serve the warm oysters with the kaffir lime sauce on the side. Enjoy!

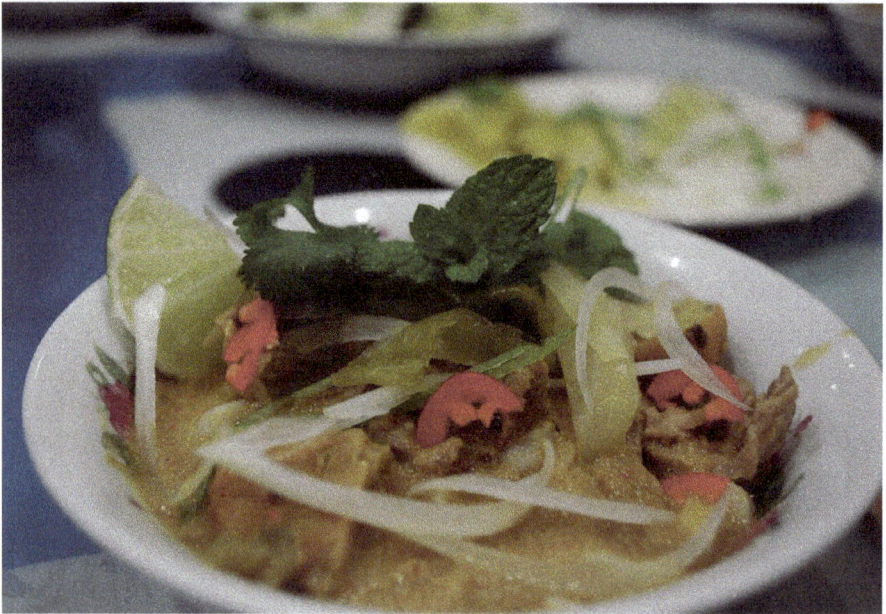

# Spicy Curried King Prawns

**Cooking Time:**

15 minutes

**Servings:**2

**Ingredients:**

12 king prawns, rinsed

1 tablespoon coconut oil

1/2 teaspoon piri piri powder

Salt and ground black pepper, to taste

1 teaspoon garlic paste

1 teaspoon onion powder

1/2 teaspoon cumin powder

1 teaspoon curry powder

**Directions:**

1.In a mixing bowl, toss all ingredient until the prawns are well coated on all sides.

2.Cook in the preheated Air Fryer at 360 degrees F for 4 minutes. Shake the basket and cook for 4 minutes more.

3.Serve over hot rice if desired. Enjoy!

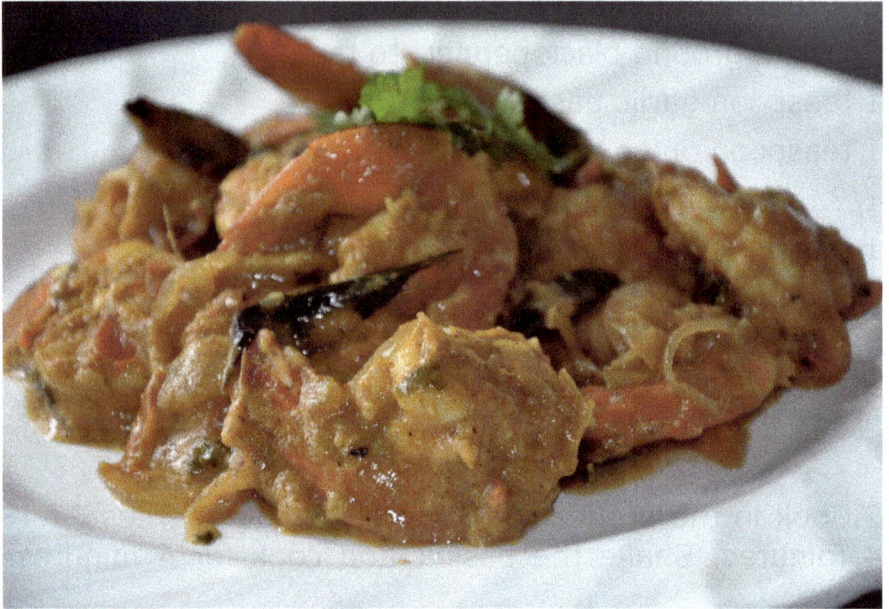

# Grilled Salmon Steaks

**Cooking Time:**

45 minutes

**Servings:**4

**Ingredients:**

2 cloves garlic, minced

4 tablespoons butter, melted

Sea salt and ground black pepper, to taste

1 teaspoon smoked paprika

1/2 teaspoon onion powder

1 tablespoon lime juice

1/4 cup dry white wine

4 salmon steaks

**Directions:**

1.Place all ingredients in a large ceramic dish. Cover and let it marinate for 30 minutes in the refrigerator. Arrange the salmon steaks on the grill pan.

2.Bake at 390 degrees for 5 minutes, or until the salmon steaks are easily flaked with a fork.

3.Flip the fish steaks, baste with the reserved marinade, and cook another 5 minutes. Serve and enjoy!

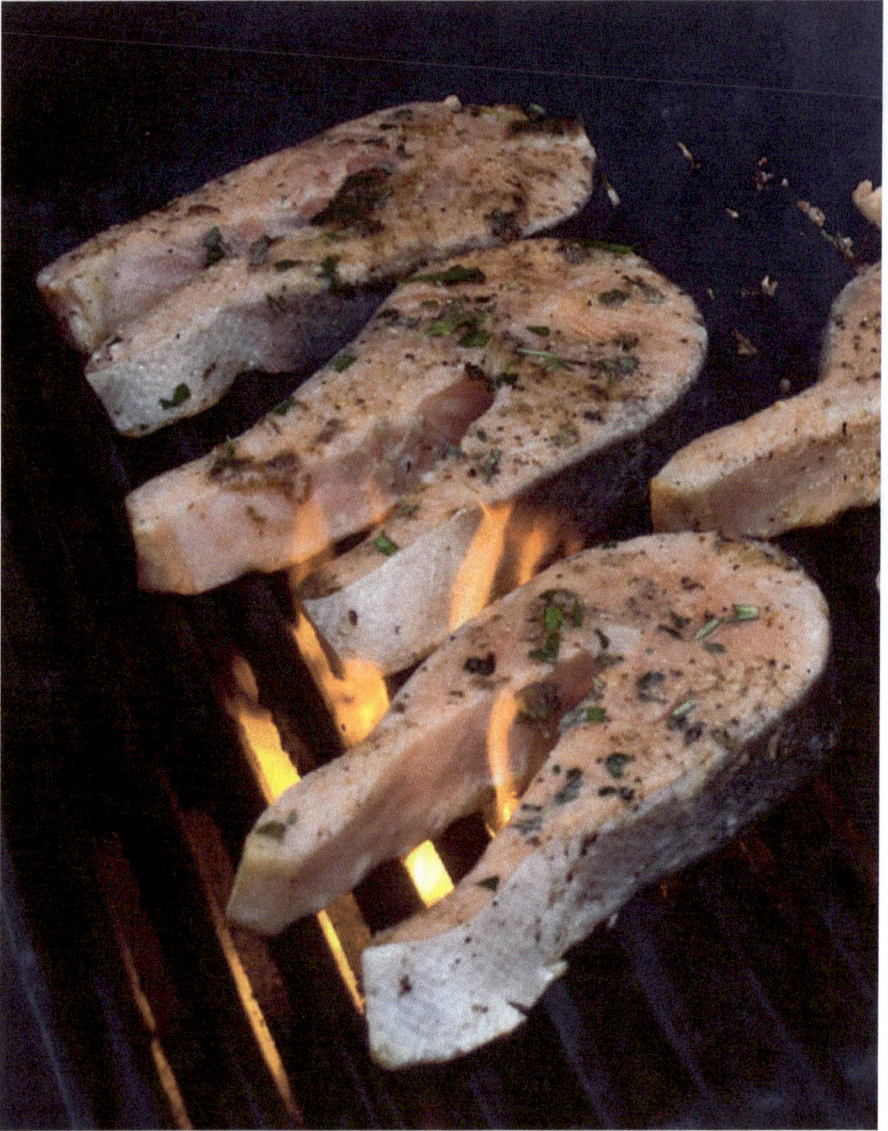

# Indian Famous Fish Curry

**Cooking Time:**

25 minutes

**Servings:**4

**Ingredients:**

2 tablespoons sunflower oil

1/2pound fish, chopped

2 red chilies, chopped

1 tablespoon coriander powder

1 teaspoon curry paste

1 cup coconut milk

Salt and white pepper, to taste

1/2 teaspoon fenugreek seeds

1 shallot, minced

1 garlic clove, minced

1 ripe tomato, pureed

**Directions:**

1.Preheat your Air Fryer to 380 degrees F; brush the cooking basket with 1 tablespoon of sunflower oil. Cook your fish for 10 minutes on both sides.

2.Transfer to the baking pan that is previously greased with the remaining tablespoon of sunflower oil.

3.Add the remaining ingredients and reduce the heat to 350 degrees F. Continue to cook an additional 10 to 12 minutes or until everything is heated through. Enjoy!

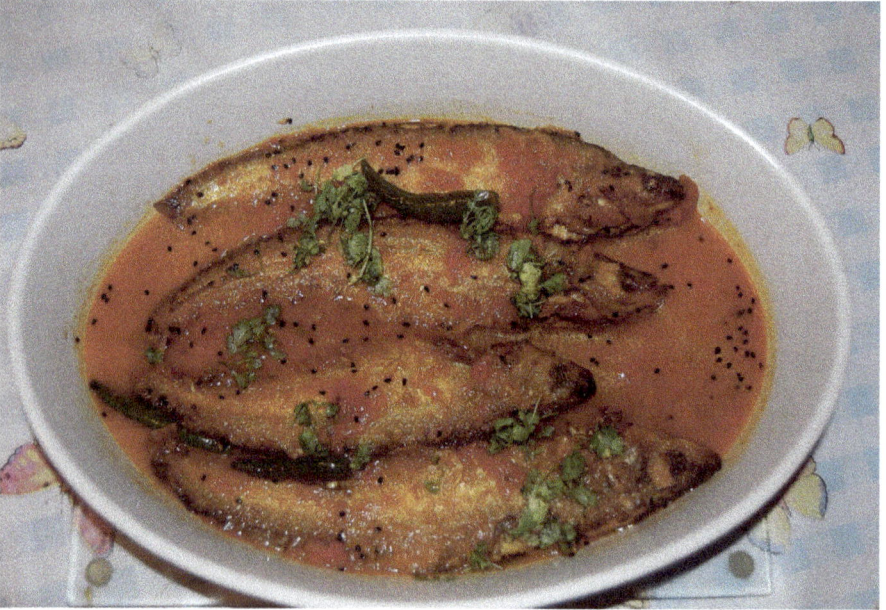

# Crispy Prawns in Bacon Wraps

**Cooking Time:**

30 minutes

**Servings:**4

**Ingredients:**

8 bacon slices

8 jumbo prawns, peeled and deveined

## *Directions:*

1.Wrap each prawn from head to tail with each bacon slice overlapping to keep the bacon in place.

2.Secure the ends with toothpicks. Refrigerate for 15 minutes. Preheat air fryer to 400 F.

3.Arrange the bacon-wrapped prawns on the greased frying basket and Bake for 8 minutes, turning once. Serve hot.

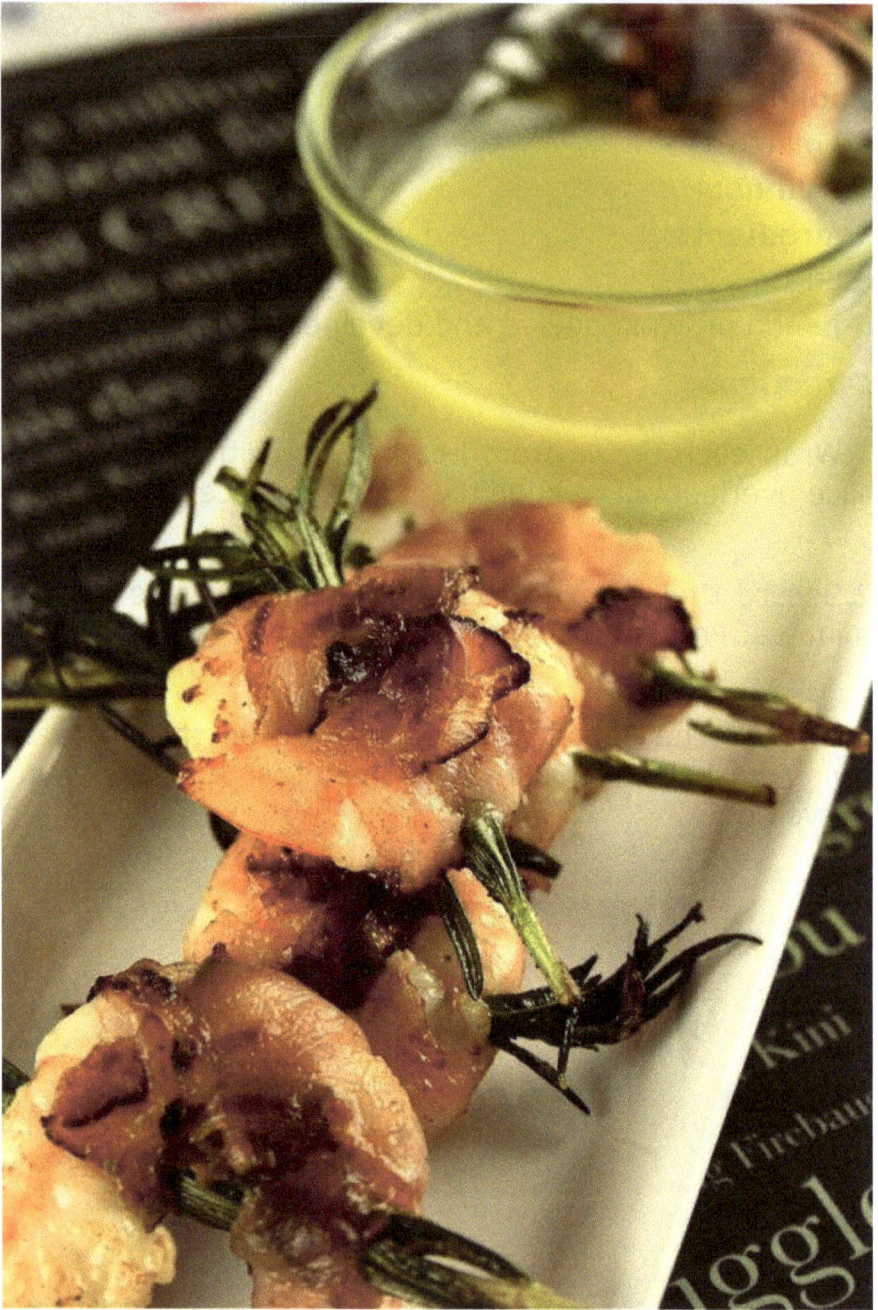

# Mango Shrimp Skewers with Hot Sauce

**Cook Time:**

20minutes

**Servings:**4

**Ingredients:**

20 small-sized shrimp, peeled and deveined

2 tbsp olive oil

½ tsp garlic powder

1 tsp mango powder

2 tbsp fresh lime juice

Salt and black pepper to taste

2 tbsp fresh cilantro, chopped

1 garlic clove, minced

1 green onion, finely sliced

1 tbsp red chili flakes, crushed

4 tbsp olive oil

2 tbsp white wine vinegar

**Directions:**

1.In a bowl, mix garlic powder, mango powder, lime juice, salt, and black pepper.

2.Add the shrimp and toss to coat. Cover and marinate for 20 minutes. Soak wooden skewers in water for 15 minutes.

3.In a small dish, mix cilantro, minced garlic, green onion, chili flakes, olive oil, and champagne vinegar. Preheat air fryer to 390 F. Thread the marinated shrimp onto the skewers, drizzle with olive oil, and place in the frying basket.

4.AirFry for 5 minutes, shake the shrimp, and cook for 5 more minutes. Serve the skewers with the cilantro sauce.

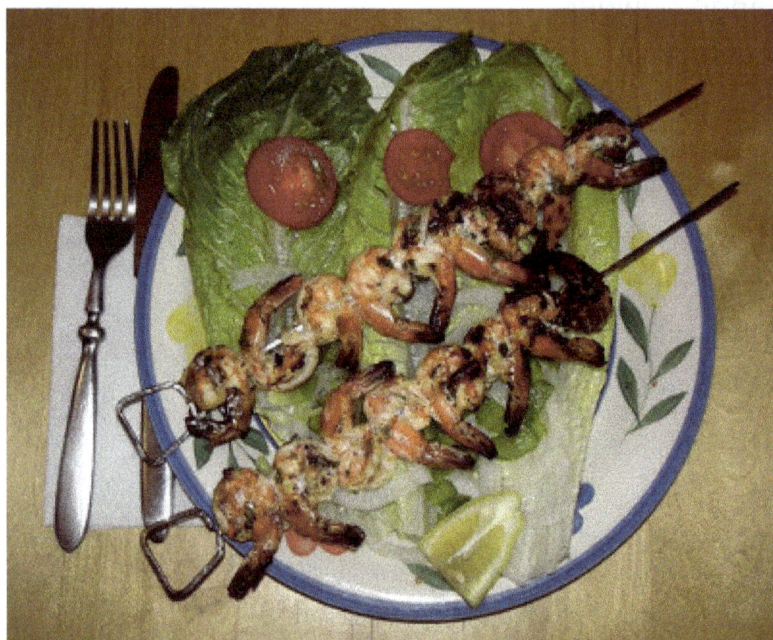

# American Panko Fish Nuggets

***Cook Time:***

*20 minutes*

***Servings:****4*

**Ingredients:**

1 lb fish fillets

1 lemon, juiced

Salt and black pepper to taste

1 tsp dried dill

4 tbsp mayonnaise

2 eggs, beaten

1 tbsp garlic powder

1 cup breadcrumbs

1 tsp paprika

**Directions:**

1Preheat air fryer to 400 F. Season the fish with salt and black pepper.

2.In a bowl, mix beaten eggs, lemon juice, and mayonnaise.

3.In a separate bowl, mix breadcrumbs, paprika, dill, and garlic powder. Dredge the fillets in the egg mixture and then in the crumbs.

4.Place the fillets in the greased frying basket and Air Fryer for 15 minutes, flipping once halfway through. Serve warm.

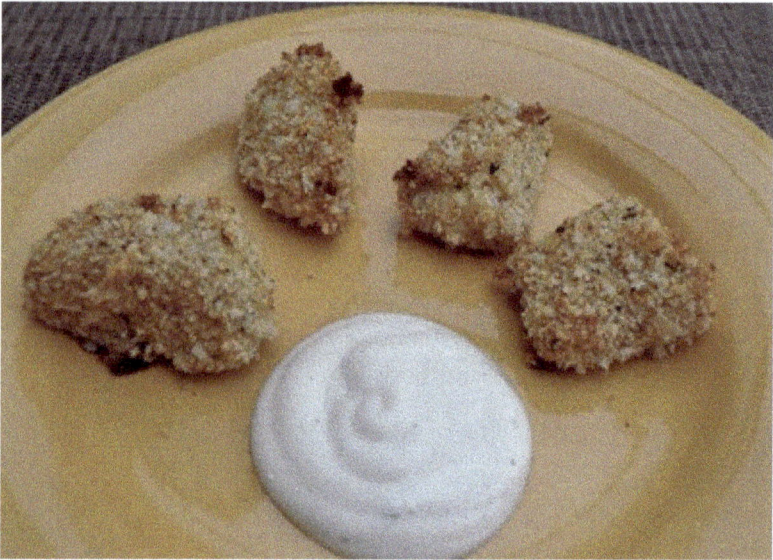

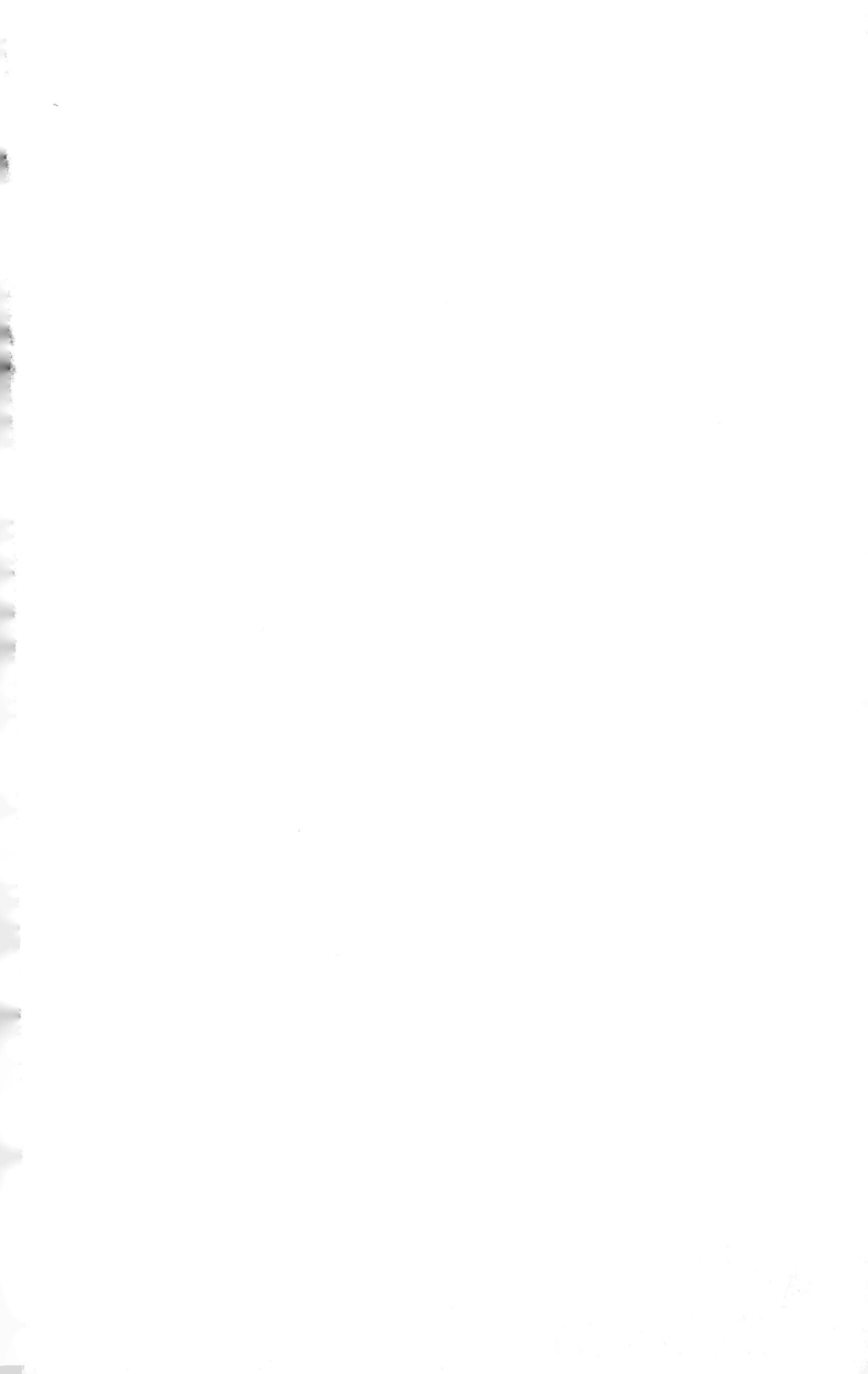

www.ingramcontent.com/pod-product-compliance
Lightning Source LLC
Chambersburg PA
CBHW050756030426
42336CB00012B/1846